PURSUITS OF HAPPINESS

D1479082

PURSUITS OF HAPPINESS

Well-Being in Anthropological Perspective

Edited by
Gordon Mathews and Carolina Izquierdo

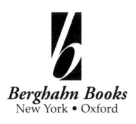

Berghahn Books
New York • Oxford

First published in 2009 by

Berghahn Books

www.berghahnbooks.com

©2009, 2010 Gordon Mathews and Carolina Izquierdo
First paperback edition published in 2010

Library of Congress Cataloging-in-Publication Data

Pursuits of happiness : well-being in anthropological perspective / edited by
Gordon Mathews and Carolina Izquierdo.
    p. cm.
    Includes bibliographical references and index.
    ISBN 978-1-84545-448-7 (hbk.)—ISBN 978-1-84545-708-2 (pbk.)
    1. Quality of life—Cross-cultural studies. 2. Well-being—Cross-cultural
studies. 3. Happiness—Cross-cultural studies. 4. Anthropology—Philosophy. I. Mathews, Gordon. II. Izquierdo, Carolina.
HN25.P87 2008
306.09—dc22
                                                                    2008028586

British Library Cataloguing in Publication Data

A catalogue record for this book is available from the British Library

Printed in the United States on acid-free paper.

ISBN: 978-1-84545-448-7 Hardback
ISBN: 978-1-84545-708-2 Paperback

Contents

List of Tables and Figures

Tables

Figures

Acknowledgements

We are grateful to Elinor Ochs, director of the Center for the Everyday Lives of Families (CELF) at UCLA. It is with her support and the funding by the Alfred P. Sloan Foundation that a 2002 workshop brought together scholars interested in well-being. An American Anthropological Association panel followed, leading, eventually, to the chapters that comprise this book. We thank Tom Weisner for his participation and help throughout the years in facilitating this book. We thank Lynne Nakano, for providing a close and perceptive reading of the book manuscript. And we thank an anonymous referee for Berghahn Books, who was enormously helpful in suggestions for the initial manuscript's revision.

List of Contributors

Naomi Adelson is Associate Professor, Department of Anthropology, York University, Toronto, Canada. She is the author of *'Being Alive Well': Health and the Politics of Cree Well-Being* (2000), as well as numerous book chapters and articles.

Scott Clark is Professor of Anthropology at the Rose-Hulman Institute of Technology, Indiana. He is a specialist in Japanese society and culture, and is the author of *Japan, a View from the Bath* (1994), as well as numerous articles.

Benjamin Nick Colby is Emeritus Professor in the Social Dynamics and Complexity Group, Institute for Mathematical Behavioral Sciences, and the Department of Anthropology at the University of California, Irvine. He is a founding editor of *Structure and Dynamics: eJournal of Anthropological and Related Sciences* and has published ethnographies on Zinacantan and the Ixil Maya.

Steve Derné is Professor of Sociology at the State University of New York–Geneseo. His research projects have examined family life, emotions, filmgoing, and globalization in India. His books are *Culture in Action: Family, Emotion, and Male Dominance in Banaras, India* (1995), *Movies, Masculinity, and Modernity: An Ethnography of Men's Filmgoing in India* (2000), and *Globalization on the Ground: Media and the Transformation of Culture, Class and Gender in India* (2008).

Daniela Heil is a Lecturer in the Department of Sociology and Anthropology, University of Newcastle, Australia. Her research (in New South Wales, southeastern Australia and the Kimberley, Western Australia) addresses the conjunctures and disjunctures of Aboriginal and "Western" understandings of "health" and "well-being." She is currently completing a book, *Well-being and Bodies in Trouble*.

Douglas Hollan is Professor and Luckman Distinguished Teacher at UCLA and instructor at the New Center for Psychoanalysis in Los Angeles. He is the author of numerous articles examining the interface of cultural and psychological processes and is co-author of *Contentment and Suffering: Culture and Experience in Toraja* (1994) and *The Thread of Life: Toraja Reflections on the Life Cycle* (1996).

Carolina Izquierdo is currently a postdoctoral researcher at the Center for the Everyday Lives of Families (CELF) at the University of California, Los Angeles. She has done extensive research on well-being among the Matsigenka in the Peruvian Amazon, among the Mapuche in Chile, and among middle-class working families in the United States.

William Jankowiak is Professor of Anthropology at the University of Nevada, Las Vegas. He is the author of *Sex, Death, and Hierarchy in a Chinese City* (1992), editor of *Romantic Passion* (1995), co-editor of *Drugs, Labor, and Colonial Expansion* (2003), and editor of *Intimacies: Love and Sex across Cultures* (2008).

Gordon Mathews is a Professor in the Department of Anthropology at the Chinese University of Hong Kong. He has written *What Makes Life Worth Living? How Japanese and Americans Make Sense of Their Worlds* (1996) and *Global Culture/Individual Identity: Searching for Home in the Cultural Supermarket* (2000), and co-written *Hong Kong, China: Learning to Belong to a Nation* (2008); he has co-edited *Consuming Hong Kong* (2001) and *Japan's Changing Generations* (2004).

Neil Thin is a Senior Lecturer in the Department of Social Anthropology, School of Social and Political Studies, University of Edinburgh. He has researched and advised on social planning in international development for twenty years, and is the author of numerous guidance books and theoretical texts on poverty and social development, including *Social Progress and Sustainable Development* (2002).

Thomas S. Weisner is Professor in the Departments of Anthropology and Psychiatry (Semel Institute) and Director, Center for Culture & Health, UCLA. His interests are in culture, human development and the family, and evidence-informed policy, in both Africa and the United States. He is the author of numerous articles, and edited *African Families and the Crisis of Social Change* (with Bradley and Kilbride) (1997), and *Discovering Successful Pathways in Children's Development* (2005). He is past president of the Society for Psychological Anthropology of the American Anthropological Association.

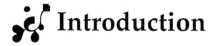
Introduction

ANTHROPOLOGY, HAPPINESS, AND WELL-BEING
Gordon Mathews and Carolina Izquierdo

Today, happiness is everywhere—at least in bookstores. There are numerous tomes to be found on "happiness," "the pursuit of happiness," "the history of happiness," and "the science of happiness," teaching, in so many words, how to become happy. Some of these books are very informative, based in evidence from the research of psychologists and economists and other experts (see, for example, Gilbert 2007; Layard 2005; McMahon 2006), but most more or less share a common misunderstanding. They assume that there is a single "pursuit of happiness"—but is there? We argue that there is not. Happiness is not one thing; it means different things in different places, different societies, and different cultural contexts. There is no unambiguously single pursuit of happiness—rather, there are multiple "pursuits of happiness."

This is where anthropology comes in. Sociocultural anthropology is primarily the study of different societies in all their social and cultural specificity and complexity. Most of the chapters of this book, based on an anthropologist's long-term experience and ethnographic research in a given society, indicate how happiness is conceived of, expressed, and experienced in that society. Thus, for example, Heil in chapter 4 shows how for the Australian Aborigines she lived with, it is a matter of being immersed in a close network of kin, in all the mutual social obligations this entails. Derné in chapter 6 shows how for young Indian men, it is a matter of being comfortably guided by one's parents in one's crucial life decisions, such as whom to marry. Jankowiak in chapter 7, by contrast, shows how for Chinese in the early 2000s, it is a matter of being able to pursue one's own freely chosen goals in life, unrestrained by government control of one's life. Clark, in chapter 9, shows how for Japanese, it may be based in the socially experienced physical pleasure of the bath. As these and many other chapters in this book imply, happiness is not necessarily the same everywhere; the experience of happiness is culturally specific.

And yet it is not only culturally specific. Today we may pick up cultural influences from far-flung societies the world over: a Mumbai businesswoman may seek happiness through a popular American self-help book, while her New York counterpart may seek happiness instead through the guidance of the *Bhagavad Gita* or a twenty-first-century Indian guru's writings. Underlying this is the fact that we are all human, sharing a broadly common physical and genetic makeup, and on that basis experiencing the world in broadly common ways. Although there are exceptions in various places and times and situations, by and large human beings the world over have preferred love over hate within their particular human group, freedom from pain over experiencing pain, and meaning over meaninglessness. Beneath all the cultural diversity in happiness, there is a stratum of human commonality—anthropology in its ethnographic portraits of particular peoples can teach us not only about their happiness, but, at least indirectly, about our own happiness as well.

And that is the purpose of this book. Most of the chapters of this book discuss specific societies, but the implications of their discussions may transcend these societies. This book's most basic argument is that by understanding happiness—or well-being—in a diverse array of societies, we can begin to understand it in its cultural specificities and also in a broader, human sense. First, however, let us set forth a change in terms. Happiness is a difficult term to discuss because it is ultimately subjective—who but a given individual can say whether she is happy or not? (As a stereotypical fragment of conversation might have it, "I think she's crazy. But if it makes her happy, what can I say?") Beyond this, in English as well as a number of other languages, what exactly "happiness" refers to between the transient and the permanent is unclear. In English, inquiries into happiness may for some evoke thoughts of a good meal, for others a nice car, for others a good marriage, and for others a good relationship with God. These different forms of happiness are not the same thing, despite being covered by a common term, and the same is the case for the equivalents to happiness in languages other than English. All in all, comparisons of happiness across societies seem problematic, due to linguistic and cultural barriers that seem impossible to fully surmount (Mathews 2006). Well-being, on the other hand, has an objective as well as subjective component. Happiness is a distinctive part of well-being, the most essential part; but well-being is more than that, which is why it is the centerpiece of this book's analysis.

The Meanings of Well-Being

What, then, is well-being? One place to begin is with the standard dictionary definition of the term: "the state of being healthy, happy, or prosperous." The "or" indicates that well-being might refer to any of these three attributes, but the fact that these three terms are placed together in the definition implies their interconnection. But what is the relation of "happy" to "healthy" and "prosperous"? "Healthy" refers to a positive state of one's body, and "prosperous" to a positive state of one's finances. Both of these may contribute to "happiness," a positive state of one's mind, but they may not: some of us know of physically healthy, financially well-off people who, in their intense unhappiness, commit suicide. These three attributes refer to positive states in different realms that may be but are not necessarily related. Nonetheless, this commonsensical definition does give a sense of what we mean when we use the term *well-being.* It connotes being well psychologically, physically, and socioeconomically, and, we should add, culturally: it is all these things working together.

The beauty of this term, for our purposes, is that it combines the objective and the subjective, enabling both the examination of happiness in what exactly it means and feels like in different cultural contexts, and also a more detached view, enabling at least the possibility of societal comparison. If we are going to explore the broadest human connotations of happiness, then that term itself should perhaps best be laid aside in favor of a broader panhuman term—one that, unlike *happiness,* may not necessarily be used by the people that anthropologists study. This term, the term we will use throughout this book, is *well-being.*

Well-being is not nearly as common a term as *happiness,* at least not in the popular literature, but it too has exploded in its usage over the past two decades, becoming an important term for social sciences such as economics, public health, and psychology, although not anthropology. The term has become widely used for a variety of reasons. One reason for its growing usage is the realization by economists that measures such as income—defining standard of living—cannot fully tell us about what makes life good or less good to live in different places. Thus they seek a broader, better measure. Another, quite different reason is that medical professionals have increasingly come to realize that merely keeping people alive, in an era in which medical technology has been rapidly developing, is insufficient; rather, individuals' well-being must also be closely considered. Another reason is that many psychologists have in recent decades turned from the study of mental illness to the study of mental health: from the study of "ill-being" to the study of well-being, and how to attain and maintain such a state. Finally, there has increasingly emerged in the United States and other affluent societies the idea that well-being is not simply to be assumed as a matter of good fortune, but must be strived for, fueling a massive self-help industry. Well-being has thus come into prominence for an array of disparate reasons in different fields. Well-being, it is now generally recognized, cannot be taken for granted, but must be studied and consciously pursued—and analyzed.

Well-being is often used interchangeably with a number of other terms. *Well-being* and *quality of life* seem almost synonymous in their usages in a range of disciplines, in such diverse areas as medicine and rehabilitation (as in the journal *Quality of Life Research*), economics, and philosophy (Ferry 2005; Nussbaum and Sen 1993). *Well-being* is also sometimes used synonymously with *wellness* and *health* (Brim et al. 2004; Bryant et al. 2001). *Well-being* is also used in a way that seems synonymous with *life satisfaction* (Bornstein et al. 2003; Diener and Suh 2000). In this book, we use *well-being* rather than *quality of life* in that the latter, in much of the literature, implies external observation and evaluation alone; *well-being,* on the other hand, also implies consideration of people's own internal states of mind. Anthropology, as we have discussed, is a discipline based in the latter more than the former; it typically seeks "to grasp the native's point of view" (Malinowski 1961 [1922], 25), rather than simply imposing an observer's view. We use *well-being* rather than *wellness* or *health,* in that the latter terms focus primarily on physical well-being, which is a necessary part of well-being but by no means encompasses the term. Indeed, as chapters in this book by Izquierdo (chapter 3) and Heil (chapter 4) reveal, health and well-being may contradict one another.

Let us now try to come up with a fuller, more exact definition of well-being. This is complicated, because different disciplines define well-being in distinctly different ways. Veenhoven, to cite a contemporary sociological authority, has discussed the various ways in which well-being is conceptualized (2004). He characterizes sociologists and economists as conceiving of well-being as "living in a good environment," while psychologists as well as healthcare professionals tend to conceive of it as being well-equipped "to cope with the problems of life" (2004, 5–6). Veenhoven writes that well-being is "a typical catch-all term without a precise meaning" (2004, 5). This seems true, and yet the broadest formulations of the term do attempt to combine the external and the internal, the objective and subjective modes that Veenhoven describes:

> Well-being is a positive state of affairs, brought about by the simultaneous satisfaction of personal, relational, and collective needs of individuals and communities (Prilleltensky 2005).

> Well-being incorporates a variety of objective factors such as being healthy, being safe (from crime or violence), being financially secure, hav-

ing access to resources, including education, culture, roads, and trans-
port. Well-being also however incorporates more subjective factors such
as being happy ... feeling connected to one's community and having the
capacity to cope with adverse life events (Ogilvie 2002).

These formulations are somewhat culture-bound, especially the second;
but they do have the merit of encompassing objective and subjective
conceptions of well-being, and interlinking the individual, community, and society in their definitions. Let us now offer our own broad
definition:

> Well-being is an optimal state for an individual, community, society, and
> the world as a whole. It is conceived of, expressed, and experienced in
> different ways by different individuals and within the cultural contexts
> of different societies: different societies may have distinctly different cul-
> turally shaped visions of well-being. Nonetheless, well-being bears a de-
> gree of commonality due to our common humanity and interrelatedness
> over space and time. Well-being is experienced by individuals—its essen-
> tial locus lies within individual subjectivity—but it may be considered
> and compared interpersonally and interculturally, since all individuals
> live within particular worlds of others, and all societies live in a common
> world at large.

Different chapters of this book offer different particular formulations
of well-being, in ethnographically portraying different social and cultural contexts, but all the chapters of the book fit within this broad
formulation.

The above formulation differs from the earlier ones we cited in its
stress on different social and cultural senses of well-being. The single
greatest lack, in the different disciplinary conceptions of well-being we
have discussed, is their refusal to examine how well-being is conceived
of differently in different social and cultural contexts across the globe.
This is what anthropology can provide: one more essential piece to the
puzzle of well-being considered worldwide. Returning to the three
terms of our earlier definition, health and prosperity can be measured
objectively by physicians, public health experts, or economists, whether
in terms of individuals or of a society at large. However, the valuation
given to these domains may differ in different societies with, for example, some societies seeing wealth as the greatest of all personal goals
and others seeing the desire for wealth as contemptible. Beyond this,
happiness, as we have argued, is subjective and culture bound, and
cannot easily be ascertained by any universal measures. Different societies may adhere to different culturally and linguistically constructed
concepts of happiness, making cross-societal comparison more or less
problematic. Even more fundamentally, different societies have differ-

ent cultural conceptions of what it means to be happy, satisfied, and well that must be taken into consideration.

Having said this, however, these different conceptions of health, wealth, and happiness are for the most part not incommensurable. Underlying these different conceptions, it is indeed possible to make a comparison of different societies as to well-being, as long as this is done in a careful, culturally sensitive way. This can be done through what we in this book term *soft comparison,* comparison based not on—or at least not solely on—bald statistics placed side by side, but rather on all the nuances of sociocultural context ethnographically portrayed. But before exploring this, let us examine recent attempts of other disciplines as to the societal comparison of well-being.

The Comparison of Different Societies as to Well-Being

Over the past several decades, the comparison of societies by NGOs and academic think tanks as to well-being has become widespread and influential. Most of these ratings are made on the basis of measurable data, in terms of, for example, per capita income, life expectancy, education levels, and rates of infant mortality. These rankings clearly rate something of importance. Many of us would rather live in a society with long life expectancy, high levels of literacy, and ready access to healthcare and clean water, than a society with low levels of these attributes. But the relation of these external markers to internal states of well-being remains an open question. Erich Fromm, in the opening chapter of his book *The Sane Society* (1955), asks how it can be that the societies with the most wealth also have the highest rates of "destructive acts" (suicide/homicide) and of alcoholism—contradictions that can be seen as much today as when Fromm wrote. Certainly many works of fiction and film depicting societies near the top of most well-being indexes, such as those of Western Europe, as well as Japan and the United States, depict all too convincingly Thoreau's famous observation that "the mass of men lead lives of quiet desperation." This point can be overstated; surveys show that "in general people in rich countries are ... happier than people in poor countries" (Frey and Stutzer 2002, 9), a point that, whatever reservations one may have about such surveys, seems plausible. But the statistical measures mentioned above leave aside the crucial matter of how people themselves feel about their lives, and without that, how much can we really understand?

Indeed, well-being, as we have formulated it, connotes subjectivity. While well-being "largely arises from and is influenced by various structural arrangements in which individuals are imbedded" (Pearlin 1989, 241)—the cultural patternings, social relations, and institutional arrangements within which we live—it is nonetheless experienced as individual. A number of psychologists have recognized this. In contrast to objective well-being, measures of health and wealth and other external factors, they investigate what they term "subjective well-being": how individuals themselves rate their well-being, in answering questions about how satisfied they are with their lives. Diener and Suh (2000), to mention one prominent example, examine in their edited book senses of subjective well-being across a range of societies, on the basis of cross-cultural survey research.

At first glance, this may seem to solve the problem of subjectivity—after all, people report on their own feelings of well-being in such surveys—but fuller consideration shows that the problem of understanding how people themselves understand their lives remains. Surveys do not ask respondents to talk about their senses of well-being in their own words. Rather, they ask for informants' closed-ended answers to fixed questions, as translated into different languages. This not only ignores how individuals express their own senses of their lives, but also ignores how different languages and cultures conceive of well-being in different ways. The problem here is that which we earlier discussed in terms of happiness: cross-cultural comparison of survey data leaves out too much to be fully credible.

Let us provide one example of this. "Why are North Americans happier than East Asians?" asks a chapter in Diener and Suh's above-cited book (Suh 2000, 64, 72). This question assumes that the survey results being compared reflect the underlying reality of happiness and well-being or the lack thereof, rather than represent the product of the surveys themselves and their culturally shaped responses. As a more skeptical observer has noted, Americans may "inflate their reports of happiness. ... Most modern Americans say they are very or extremely happy, and one must be skeptical about whether their lives are really so wonderful" as the quick answers they give to survey questions indicate (Baumeister 1991, 210). Indeed, in a society declaring in its founding document the inalienable right to "the pursuit of happiness," one is culturally enjoined to pursue and proclaim one's happiness. It is almost as if one is required to be happy, or at least to be able to describe how one is earnestly pursuing such a state, in order to be fully and normally American. In East Asian societies such as Japan, on the other hand, personal modesty is an ingrained social value—one is enjoined not to boast about one's success in life or declare too loudly one's personal happiness or well-being. To proclaim happiness, even in an anonymous survey, may be felt to be an affront to modesty. Thus it may well be that North Americans are not "happier than Asians," but are simply more willing to proclaim their happiness on a survey form.[1]

This is not to dismiss all survey research, some of which can indeed be valuable. As earlier noted, measures such as life expectancy, infant mortality, literacy rates, and per capita income are important in understanding a society's senses of well-being. Findings concerning "subjective well-being" may also be quite useful in some contexts (see, as one interesting example, Helliwell 2002). The problem remains, however, that none of these measures, of objective well-being or of subjective well-being, can fully get at well-being in all its complexity. For this kind of examination, we must turn to anthropology, the empirical study of culture. This book will show how anthropology can particularly contribute to the analysis of societies as to well-being, and thereby lend a greater degree of nuance to the cross-cultural comparison of well-being.

Anthropology and the Study of Well-Being

While economists, public health specialists, and psychologists as well as other social scientists have written many books and articles on well-being and have been widely influential in their findings, anthropologists have been almost entirely silent. Anthropologists sometimes make use of comparative statistical measures such as life expectancy, but are usually unwilling to generalize about well-being on the basis of such measures. Anthropologists also tend to be highly skeptical of psychological surveys such as those we have discussed, seeing them as inevitably ethnocentric in their use of Western-derived survey instruments to compare a range of societies across the world. While these psychological studies are becoming more sophisticated, taking into account cultural differences in conception and expression (see the review of well-being research by Diener and Tov 2007[2]), many anthropologists remain dubious. After all, the very act of measurement presumes a common cross-cultural scale; but is there any such scale? Doesn't any effort to create such a scale inevitably privilege some cultural conceptions over others? And doesn't it reify what can be measured, and ignore what cannot be measured? Many would answer these last two questions with a clear "yes."

Some anthropologists, such as Colby in chapter 2 of this book, argue that these difficulties can be overcome, enabling cross-cultural statistical comparison; chapters 1 and 2 both offer arguments that support, on very different bases, the broad-based cross-cultural comparison of well-being. However, most anthropologists, including most of those appearing in the remaining chapters of this book, are skeptical of such efforts. Indeed, the reader will find that one function of this book as a whole is to show that the American or Western conceptions of well-being are insufficient to understand well-being in a range of societies across the globe, and are thus insufficient as a basis for the cross-cultural comparison of well-being.

Anthropologists specialize in understanding, through extended fieldwork, the complex cultural meanings that exist within a given society. They may be especially well situated to understand a given society's particular linguistic formulations of well-being and to reveal, through close ethnographic description, how these play out in people's daily lives, words, and worlds. Although the term *well-being* has been little used among anthropologists until recently (see Colby 1987; Adelson 2000), many anthropologists have, in effect, engaged in the study of well-being in their meticulous ethnographies. To name just a few of many, Schieffelin's (1976) discussion of Kaluli existential perceptions of life as expressed in ceremony, Bourgois's (1995) account of life in a New York City crack den, Plath's (1980) account of the meaning of maturity in modern Japan, and Whyte's (1997) explication of how misfortune is made sense of in Uganda are all very complex discussions of well-being and what it means in different social milieu, despite the fact that these books hardly use the term.

Why are anthropologists so leery of examining well-being? Thin fully explores this question in chapter 1, but let us offer a preliminary answer here. Largely this is because well-being, as an analytic rather than an ethnographic term, tends to be used much more by social scientists than by a given people themselves in describing their lives; but it is the latter that anthropologists have generally focused upon in their ethnographic portrayals. Many anthropologists have tended to shy away from cultural comparison and evaluation, insisting on respect for the values of a particular people, and arguing that the values and meanings of any sociocultural system should be seen in their own context. Thus, anthropologists may simply dismiss the study of well-being. This position is understandable, but in effect it renders anthropologists no more than naysayers. Economists, public health specialists, and psychologists engage in the cross-cultural comparison of well-being, however flawed their modes of comparison may be. If anthropologists merely say that such comparison is impossible and add nothing to the cross-cultural examination of well-being, then they are shutting themselves off from the effort to create cross-cultural comparisons of well-being. This is despite the fact that the complex local knowledge of anthropologists could make such comparisons more nuanced and thus more valid.

Underlying the anthropological emphasis on ethnography in all its specifics is the discipline's long history of cultural relativism. Cultural relativism is the belief that societies should not be evaluated in terms of a transcultural scale of evaluation, but taken on their own unique terms. As Melville Herskovits, a leading anthropological theorist of cultural relativism, once wrote, "there is no way to play this game of making judgments across cultures except with loaded dice" (1958, 270; quoted in Perry 2003, 169). This attitude is engrained in anthropology; introductory anthropology classes often advocate cultural relativism as an ultimate value, with ethnocentrism and judgment of other societies' cultures seen as the greatest of anthropological evils. In the late 1980s and 1990s, postmodernism took this view even further, arguing, in at least some scholars' views, that it is impossible to understand anything that occurs outside one's own culture: "the other" is impenetrably other, and objective knowledge is but a delusion.

There has been a minority of anthropologists who do engage in extensive cross-cultural research, focusing not on cultural difference but on human universals (Brown 1991). But as earlier noted, most anthropologists do not use experience-far concepts purporting to be universal, but instead use experience-near concepts in their analyses, the concepts used by their informants. This affects the anthropological analysis of well-being. Societies studied by anthropologists may have no concept of well-being, and the term may make no sense to the members of such societies. Instead, there may be a native term with different resonances, as several of the chapters of this book reveal, or no term at all. Anthropologists who study well-being may need, at least to some extent, to go beyond cultural relativism; they need at least implicitly a comparative perspective to make their analysis of well-being possible. But this has been far from the anthropological mainstream.

However, as previously mentioned, anthropologists have not been entirely absent from the topic of well-being, and have discussed issues of human well-being and ill-being. One example is Robert Edgerton, who writes in his book *Sick Societies* (1992) about groups of people who fail to survive as populations, who have harmful institutions, and whose practices impair their physical and mental health. Although Edgerton is not discussing well-being for the societies he examines, he explores in great detail what makes a population "sick." He concludes that "the ability to distinguish what is harmful for human beings from what is beneficial to them should qualify as useful knowledge" (1992, 208), and that anthropology should produce such knowledge and such evaluation. Another anthropologist who has considered issues of evaluation is Elvin Hatch, in his *Culture and Morality* (1983). Hatch writes: "Human well-being is not a culture-bound idea. ... Starvation and violence are phenomena that are recognized as such in the most diverse cultural traditions" (1983, 134). He argues for a humanistic principle that transcends cultural relativism: "We can judge that human sacrifice, torture, and political repression are wrong, whether they occur in our society or some other. Similarly, it is wrong for a person, whatever society he or she may belong to, to be indifferent towards the suffering of others" (1983, 135). Hatch acknowledges that his humanistic principle may be difficult to tightly define, but argues steadfastly for its existence, and the moral necessity for applying it.

Some anthropologists have been seen, however, as going to an extreme in their judgments; we may recall the writings of Colin Turnbull on the Ik (1972), in which he recounts with horror the various cruelties they inflicted upon one another. Appalled by the "nature" of this mountain people in Uganda, he recommended to the Ugandan government that the "ruthless," "loveless," and "miserable" Ik be relocated so that they would not starve to death, but also would not reproduce such an undesirable society. Many anthropologists reacted with outrage to such recommendations; indeed, most anthropologists have been extremely reluctant to write about the people they study in ways that could be construed as evaluations.

There also have been subdisciplines of anthropology that have specifically dealt with issues relating to well-being: these include psychological anthropology and medical anthropology. In the 1930s, 1940s, and 1950s the Culture and Personality movement (which in the 1960s became known as psychological anthropology) came under fire, for it sought to characterize entire cultures and nations according to the personality types they exhibited, sometimes in effect pathologizing other cultures despite the cultural relativistic framework in which they wrote (Benedict 1934; Kardiner 1945). For example, Benedict characterized the Dobuans of Melanesia as "paranoid," the Pueblos as "Apollonian," and the Kwakiutl as "megalomaniacal." After much criticism based on the perceived lack of objectivity of research using psychiatric terms to characterize entire populations (see Spiro 1951; Shweder 1991), this paradigm lost much of its credibility. Shweder notes that "there is no reason to expect that the ways individuals differ from one another within any or all cultures have anything to do with the ways cultures differ from one another" (1991, 292)—differences between cultures are far more complex than these simple labels allowed. More careful comparative projects subsequently emerged, such as the Whitings with their *Chil-*

dren of Six Cultures project (1963, 1975), Edgerton (1971), and Korbin (1981)—studies that maintained a cross-cultural focus dealing with topics such as child abuse, birthing practices, and mental retardation. However, despite this research, which had extensive implications for the study of well-being, interest in cross-cultural research lost many of its followers and psychological anthropologists turned instead to such topics as shamanism, emotion, and cognition, as well as mental illness and pathology (Kleinman 1980).

More recently, another more specific approach within medical anthropology has begun to question the "underlying ideological assumptions of health," addressing topics related to the cultural constructions of health that, in turn, set parameters for ideas about well-being (Adelson 2000; Blaxter 2004; Izquierdo 2005). Just as there are many ways in which well-being can be defined and measured, health is also culturally dependent. While objective measures are generally used in defining and measuring health, researchers recently have started to understand that subjective perceptions of a person's life circumstances have a stronger impact than straightforward external circumstance: "The important factor in determining happiness … is not how healthy you are, objectively, but rather how you feel about your health" (Baumeister 1991, 213).

This book represents the first time that anthropologists studying well-being in societies across the globe have been placed within the pages of a single volume; as such, it represents something new in the discipline. Most of its contributors are wedded to ethnography, and do not believe that anthropologists should offer wide-ranging moral judgments of societies. However, its contributors do believe that well-being can be ethnographically examined in a given society, and many believe that it can to some extent be compared across societies: not through "hard comparison," the statistical data of psychologists and economists and others, but through "soft comparison," on the basis of ethnography.

The Chapters of This Book

Part One of this book offers two chapters broadly theorizing well-being and societal comparison as to well-being; Parts Two, Three, and Four turn to ethnography. Part Two's three chapters consider well-being in small-scale societies on three continents, each facing the impact of the national state and of globalization. Part Three's three chapters examine well-being in India, China, and Japan between state and culture, and between living for one's group and living for oneself. Part Four's three chapters offer new frameworks for investigation, considering well-being physically, phenomenologically, and familially in Japan, Indonesia, and the United States.

This book includes contributions by many of the anthropologists in the world today working on the topic of well-being. They do not all speak in a unified voice. The book's chapters are notable for their diversity, not only in the societies they examine, but also in their differing ethnographic approaches to well-being. In particular, the theoreticians of Part One advocate the explicit comparison of societies as to well-being, a comparison that many of the ethnographers in Parts Two, Three, and Four do not fully believe in and do not practice. These ethnographic chapters themselves examine well-being from different vantage points, in accordance with the cultural concerns of the societies being examined, as well as the investigative interests of the anthropologist; they too are sometimes in implicit or explicit disagreement.

This book thus seeks not to set forth a programmatic schema for the investigation of well-being, which would be impossible given the current state of the field, but rather to open up new ground for the anthropological consideration of well-being as a valid and worthwhile topic to explore, both ethnographically and cross-culturally. This book seeks not to win converts to any particular research agenda, but rather to start conversations and get students and teachers of anthropology to think about a new area of investigation that is highly promising. The different viewpoints expressed in this book's chapters are intended to bring anthropological readers to think about the investigation of well-being in diverse ways, one or many of which may have relevance to their own research agendas. The diversity of approaches and viewpoints in this book is a strength of anthropology, we argue, in enabling well-being to be approached in a variety of ways, "stretching the investigative envelope" in contrast to the more codified and narrower approaches of other disciplines. We maintain that these different approaches and viewpoints can enable well-being to be more fully and complexly understood than it generally is at present.

Let us describe the chapters of this book in more detail. Part One offers a theoretical background to the anthropological study of well-being. It begins with Neil Thin in chapter 1 asking, "Why has anthropology ignored the study of well-being?" He explores the various reasons for this anthropological resistance, semantically parses the meanings of well-being in anthropological investigation, and then shows how the study of well-being can contribute to multiple areas of anthropology, arguing that anthropologists should explicitly engage in cross-cultural comparison in order to help make the world a better place. Chapter 2, by Benjamin Nick Colby, asks, "Is a cross-cultural measure of well-being possible or even desirable?" concluding that it is indeed possible and desirable. He goes through a litany of reasons why anthropologists have avoided such a measure, and counters each of them in his arguments, emphasizing the idea that what is to be compared is not "cultures" but rather "self-world." Finally he offers a theoretical basis for the cross-cultural statistical measurement of "adaptive potential," his conceptualization of well-being. These two chapters offer moral and empirical arguments for the anthropological assessment and comparison of well-being. While the chapters in the remainder of this book offer a different approach, eschewing the "hard" comparison of societies as to well-being and practicing instead "soft" ethnographic examination, these two chapters do set the stage for the chapters to come, in giving broad and perceptive analyses of the relation of anthropology to well-being. These authors convincingly set forth the need for the study of well-being in anthropology, even if the particular paths into well-being that they advocate are roads not taken by the books' other authors.

The book's subsequent chapters, ethnographic in focus, begin in Part Two by exploring well-being in small-scale societies. Chapter 3, by Carolina Izquierdo, analyzes well-being among the Matsigenka of the Peruvian Amazon, considering how they conceive of well-being and struggle to maintain well-being in the face of the increasing encroachment of the outside world upon their lives, including the Peruvian state and especially multinational oil companies. She notes how, despite the fact that the Matsigenka's physical health is getting better by objective indicators, their senses of well-being are in drastic decline, as evidenced by an upturn in accusations of sorcery and a general fear of the future. Daniela Heil's chapter 4 considers well-being in an Australian Aboriginal community, looking at how people in that community formulate well-being in terms of their relationships with kin and immersion in networks of social obligations and responsibilities: this is described by the terms "being well," and also being "one of us." Heil contrasts the Australian government's individualistic concept of well-being with the Aborigines' relational concept of well-being, depicting the latter as a critique of the former. Chapter 5, by Naomi Adelson, explores the ways in which well-being among the Cree of northern Canada are both grounded in traditional beliefs and activities and changing with changing times. She argues that expressions of well-being are intrinsically tied to concepts of land, literally and symbolically, in Cree lives, but she also explores how the Cree are reinventing their senses of identity and also their senses of well-being as their society is transformed through increasing linkages to the outside world and the changing of generations.

These three chapters of Part Two show small-scale societies suffering through and responding to differing degrees of encroachment by the nation and world at large. Judging from these chapters, their different senses of well-being depend in large part on the degree of cultural autonomy they feel they can maintain in the face of this encroachment.

We then turn, in Part Three, to nation-states and their citizens between culture and state and between individual and group. Steve Derné, in chapter 6, examines well-being among young, middle-class Indian men, and finds that it is fundamentally based in a sociocentric cultural orientation, whereby young men would rather be guided by their fathers in their choice of marriage partner than make such choices on their own, apart from familial guidance. This orientation, based in Indian social structure, has been challenged by globalization, but remains intact, he finds. In chapter 7, William Jankowiak considers well-being between culture and the state in China, examining how Chinese senses of well-being have been transformed in the past twenty years, as the governing ideology has shifted from communism to capitalism. He finds that there has been an extraordinary increase in well-being, because of the expansions of the horizons of individual choice among the Chinese he interviewed, which most, although not all, experienced as a personal liberation. Chapter 8, by Gordon Mathews, looks at the Japanese term *ikigai*—"that which makes life worth living"—exploring its competing meanings in Japan in recent years, connoting both "living for one's group" and "living for oneself." He then defines it as a cross-cultural marker of well-being, and uses it to examine and compare the cultural formulations, social negotiations, and institutional channeling of the pursuit of a life worth living in Japan, the United States, and Hong Kong.

Several of the chapters of Part Three seem to contradict one another. While Derné's Indian male informants desire not individual choice but familial guidance, Jankowiak's Chinese informants rejoice at their newfound individual freedom. But comparing these chapters in more depth, we see that well-being as experienced within one's group or within oneself is not only a matter of different cultural orientations in different societies, but also of state policies molding citizens in various ways. It is also a matter of universality, with human beings requiring both individual freedom and social relatedness in different social contexts, as these three chapters reveal in different ways.

We then turn, in Part Four, to new anthropological directions and frameworks for the examination of aspects of well-being in different societies. Chapter 9, by Scott Clark, considers well-being and physical pleasure in the context of the Japanese bath. He considers pleasure individually and universally, but focuses particularly on "the cultural context of pleasure" through the settings, activities, and meanings involved in "bathing-Japanese." Some aspects of this, he argues, can be experienced by outsiders, but other aspects can only be experienced by one fully immersed in the Japanese cultural context. In any case, anthropological analysis can enable a cross-cultural understanding of the cultural shaping of pleasure, he argues. Chapter 10, by Douglas Hollan, discusses well-being as contingent and subjective; it is experienced at the level of the individual on the basis of unconscious processes and the continual mapping of representations of one's past onto the sociocultural world of one's present. Hollan defines this as "selfscape," and thinks of well-being as the fit between selfscape and the physical and social world. He fleshes out these ideas in his portrayal of the selfscape of a Toraja man in highland Sulawesi, Indonesia, over the course of a day, in his familial ease as well as his fear of enemies and of magical attack. In chapter 11, Thomas S. Weisner examines well-being and family routines among American families with children with disabilities. Weisner defines well-being as "engaged participation in everyday cultural activities that are deemed desirable by a community." He sees as key to well-being the idea of sustainability, the ability to continue routines despite the difficulties that may confront these families, as shown in his ethnographic vignettes. These three chapters present three different theoretical approaches and frameworks for the examination of well-being in contemporary societies—through physical pleasure, socially experienced, through the individual lifeworlds of selves in social worlds, and through the analysis of familial routines. While their approaches are culturally particular, they can be used in ways that transcend that particularity. These final three chapters point to the ethnographically based cross-cultural analysis of aspects of well-being.

The Conclusion sums up this book's efforts: what can this book contribute to the examination of well-being? It outlines the arguments and questions raised by each of its four sections, and explores the "soft comparison" that the book's ethnographic chapters offer, detailing how far such comparison might proceed. It also offers a preliminary framework for the examination of well-being, based on the physical dimension, the interpersonal dimension, and the existential dimension of human social life, as impacted by the national and global dimension. The primary value of this book, the Conclusion argues, lies in the ethnographic particularities of its chapters, showing the complex varieties of well-being that exist around the world. But beyond this, the book's concluding pages map these varieties onto a common human framework, and point to at least the possibility of a broader, perhaps universal comparison of well-being.

Notes

1. Veenhoven (in personal conversation with Mathews) has said that in his own and others' survey research on happiness, statistical analysis reveals that only a small degree ("no more than 20 percent") of variation between societies can be attributed to cultural factors. While we certainly do not claim that culture is everything—it is one of a number of important factors shaping well-being—to use survey results that may be culturally problematic to demonstrate that culture does not matter leads to the diminution of culture as a foregone conclusion. The situation is like that of the joke about a man searching for his car keys at night. He is asked, "Where did you lose them?" and points into the blackness: "Over there." "Well, why are you looking for them here?" "The light's better here." This is said with all due respect to Veenhoven, whose sociological contribution to the study of well-being and happiness has been enormous.
2. As Diener and Tov say in their review's abstract (2007, 691), "Well-being can be understood to some degree in universal terms, but must also be understood within the framework of each culture. ... There are pancultural experiences of SWB [subjective well-being] that can be compared across cultures, but ... there are also culture-specific patterns that make cultures unique in their experience of well-being." In this statement, unlike statements by psychologists in earlier publications, the authors sound similar to anthropologists in their arguments.

References

Adelson, Naomi. 2000. *"Being Alive Well": Health and the Politics of Cree Well-Being.* Toronto: University of Toronto Press.

Baumeister, Roy F. 1991. *Meanings of Life.* New York: Guilford.

Benedict, Ruth. 1934. *Patterns of Culture.* Boston: Houghton Mifflin.

Blaxter, Mildred. 2004. *Health.* Cambridge: Polity.

Bornstein, Marc H., Lucy Davidson, Corey L. M. Keyes, and Kristin A. Moore. 2003. *Well-Being: Positive Development Across the Life Course.* Mahwah, NJ: Laurence Erlbaum Associates.

Bourgois, Philippe. 1995. *In Search of Respect: Selling Crack in El Barrio.* Cambridge: Cambridge University Press.

Brim, Orville G., Carol D. Ryff, and Ronald C. Kessler. 2004. *How Healthy Are We?: A National Study of Well-Being at Midlife.* Chicago: University of Chicago Press.

Bryant, Lucinda L., Kitty K. Corbett, and Jean S. Kutner. 2001. "In Their Own Words: A Model of Healthy Aging." *Social Science and Medicine* 53: 927–41.

Brown, Donald E. 1991. *Human Universals.* Philadelphia: Temple University Press.

Colby, Benjamin N. 1987. "Well-Being: A Theoretical Program." *American Anthropologist* 89 (4): 879–95.

Diener, Ed and Eunkook M. Suh, eds. 2000. *Culture and Subjective Well-Being.* Cambridge, MA: MIT Press.

Diener, Ed and William Tov. 2007. "Culture and Subjective Well-Being." In *Handbook of Cultural Psychology,* ed. Shinobu Kitayama and Dov Cohen, 691–713. New York: Guilford Press.

Edgerton, Robert. 1971. *The Individual in Cultural Adaptation: A Study of Four East African Societies.* Los Angeles: University of California Press.

———. 1992. *Sick Societies: Challenging the Myth of Primitive Harmony.* New York: Free Press.

Ferry, Luc. 2005. *What is the Good Life?* Trans. Lydia G. Cochrane. Chicago: University of Chicago Press.

Frey, Bruno S. and Alois Stutzer. 2002. *Happiness and Economics: How the Economy and Institutions Affect Well-Being.* Princeton, NJ: Princeton University Press.

Fromm, Erich. 1955. *The Sane Society.* Greenwich, CT: Fawcett.

Gilbert, Daniel. 2007. *Stumbling on Happiness.* New York: Vintage.

Hatch, Elvin. 1983. *Culture and Morality: The Relativity of Values in Anthropology.* New York: Columbia University Press.

Helliwell, John F. 2002. *Globalization and Well-Being.* Vancouver: University of British Columbia Press.

Herskovits, Melville. 1958. "Some Further Comments on Cultural Relativism." *American Anthropologist* 60: 266–73.

Izquierdo, Carolina. 2005. "When 'Health' is Not Enough: Societal, Individual and Biomedical Assessments of Well-being among the Matsigenka of the Peruvian Amazon." *Social Science and Medicine* 61: 727–83.

Kardiner, Abraham. 1945. *The Psychological Frontiers of Society.* New York: Columbia University Press.

Kleinman, Arthur. 1980. *Patients and Healers in the Context of Culture.* Berkeley: University of California Press.

Korbin, Jill E., ed. 1981. *Child Abuse and Neglect: Cross Cultural Perspectives.* Berkeley: University of California Press.

Layard, Richard. 2005. *Happiness: Lessons from a New Science.* London: Penguin.

Malinowski, Bronislaw. 1961 [1922]. *Argonauts of the Western Pacific.* Prospect Heights, IL: Waveland Press.

Mathews, Gordon. 2006. "Happiness and the Pursuit of a Life Worth Living: An Anthropological Approach." In *Happiness and Public Policy: Theory, Case Studies, and Implications,* ed. Y. K. Ng and L. S. Ho, 147–168. New York: Palgrave MacMillan.

McMahon, Darrin M. 2006. *Happiness: A History.* New York: Atlantic Monthly Press.

Nussbaum, Martha and Amartya Sen. 1993. *The Quality of Life.* Oxford: Clarendon.

Ogilvie, Emma. 2002. "Children and Young People in Queensland: A Snap Shot." http://www.childcomm.qld.gov.au/pdf/publications/ speeches/speeches_02/ emma_snapshot2002.pdf. Accessed 27 May 2006.

Pearlin, L. I. 1989. "The Sociological Study of Stress." *Journal of Health and Social Behavior* 30: 241–56.

Perry, Richard. 2003. *Five Key Concepts in Anthropological Thinking.* Upper Saddle River, NJ: Prentice Hall.

Plath, David W. 1980. *Long Engagements: Maturity in Modern Japan.* Stanford: Stanford University Press.

Prilleltensky, Isaac. 2005. "In Pursuit of Justice and Well-Being: Critical Approaches to Physical and Mental Health." http://www.uib.no/isf/people/doc/prilleltensky/part1/prilleltensky1.ppt. Accessed 28 Oct 2007.

Scheiffelin, Edward L. 1976. *The Sorrow of the Lonely and the Burning of the Dancers.* New York: St. Martin's Press.

Shweder, Richard A. 1991. *Thinking Through Cultures: Expeditions in Cultural Psychology.* Cambridge, MA: Harvard University Press.

Spiro, Melford E. 1951. "Culture and Personality: The National History of a False Dichotomy." *Psychiatry* 14: 19–46.

Suh, Eunkook M. 2000. "Self, the Hyphen Between Culture and Subjective Well-Being." In *Culture and Subjective Well-Being,* ed. Ed Diener and Eunkook M. Suh, 61–86. Cambridge, MA: MIT Press.

Turnbull, Collin. 1972. *The Mountain People.* New York: Simon & Schuster.

Veenhoven, Ruut. 2004. "Subjective Measures of Well-Being." Discussion Paper No. 2004/07, United Nations University. http://www.ciaonet.org/wps/ver01/. Accessed 23 June 2005.

Whiting, Beatrice B., ed. 1963. *Six Cultures: Studies of Child Rearing.* New York: John Wiley.

Whiting, Beatrice Blyth and John W. M. Whiting. 1975. *Children of Six Cultures: A Psycho-cultural Analysis.* Cambridge, MA: Harvard University Press.

Whyte, Susan Reynolds. 1997. *Questioning Misfortune: The Pragmatics of Uncertainty in Eastern Uganda.* Cambridge: Cambridge University Press.

PART ONE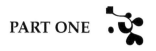

THEORETICAL BACKGROUND

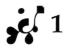 1

Why Anthropology Can Ill Afford to Ignore Well-Being

Neil Thin

> The goal [of ethnography] … is, briefly, to grasp the native's point of view, his relation to life, to realize his vision of his world … what concerns him most intimately, that is, the hold which life has on him. In each culture, the values are slightly different; people aspire after different aims, follow different impulses, yearn after a different form of happiness. To study the institutions, customs, and codes or to study the behavior and mentality without the subjective desire of feeling by what these people live, of realizing the substance of their happiness … is … to miss the greatest reward which we can hope to obtain from the study of man.
>
> Malinowski 1978 [1922], 25.

In his foundational text, Malinowski urged anthropologists to explore diverse views on happiness and the meaning of life. Imagine how you would feel if, similarly assuming sociocultural anthropology to be about things that humans care about, your proposals to study well-being received the following advice from colleagues:

> "That doesn't sound very anthropological: it's too individualistic and psychological. Not to mention ethnocentric and value-laden. We study relations, structures, and networks, not motives and feelings. We don't make evaluative judgments."

> "If you must explore psychology, avoid emotions and stick with cognitive psychology: explore mental maps, terminologies, and symbolic patterning, but not motives and feelings."

> "If you do look at emotions, focus on collective representations of these — rituals and language, not private experience."

> "If you still insist that emotional experience matters, dwell on the *adverse* emotions. Look at anger, hate, suffering, depression, fear, shame and embarrassment. Give love, aspiration, joy, and satisfaction a wide berth."

> "If you're still insistent on 'well-being,' you could treat it as a health issue, or use it as a heading but actually write about the things that go horribly wrong with people's lives."

Exaggerated though this may sound, academic social anthropology does seem to have been imbibing this kind of advice despite Malinowski's initial pleas. Sociocultural anthropology has been institutionally averse to the study of well-being. In his introductory textbook, Eriksen briefly alludes to the discipline's recent and marginal interest in the emotions, noting that "many anthropologists still take them more or less for granted and presume that they are inborn." Next, he notes the rise since the 1970s of attention to the "social construction of emotions" (1995, 227). The implication? Only when recognized as "socially constructed" are the emotions deemed worthy of anthropological study.

Though no serious anthropologist could deny that emotions are *both* inborn *and* products of cultural learning and social construction, and both private and public, in practice most anthropologists have treated them as natural and private, and therefore irrelevant to social analysis. We have been particularly reluctant to address *subjective* well-being, the experience of feeling happy, which is arguably how most humans feel most of the time (Diener and Diener 1996). Anthropologists have been far more interested in pathologies and oddities than in normality. Yet a responsible exploration of the human condition, surely, must from the outset offer some basic description of normal happiness. We could then try to interpret the great wonder of this almost universal achievement. How is well-being achieved, by different kinds of people, at various stages in their lives, in diverse contexts, despite the ever-threatening sources of harm and misery? Are these achievements really as uninteresting as Tolstoy implied in his brash opening of *Anna Karenina*: "Happy families are all alike; every unhappy family is unhappy in its own way"?

Clearly meant as a teaser, Tolstoy's aphorism is often quoted as an intellectual sneer at the banality of happiness. Most anthropologists have similarly assumed well-being to be too boringly uniform to merit attention. Exceptions have largely been confined to the "lost Eden" myths that tell us how happy or affluent people were until modernity started spoiling everything. Famous examples of naïve romanticism and anti-developmentalism include Lévi-Strauss's claim in *Tristes Tropiques* that it "would have been better for our well-being" if mankind had stayed in the Neolithic stage of evolution (1973 [1955], 446); Lorna Marshall's book *The Harmless People* (1959), which portrayed the !Kung as happy and peace-loving, overlooking the appalling rates of !Kung-!Kung violence and murder; Turnbull's *The Forest People* which portrayed Mbuti life as "a wonderful thing full of joy and happiness and free of care" in which people remained blissfully insouciant towards the hardships and dangers of the forest (1961, 29); Sahlins's "Original Affluent Society" essay, claiming that hunter-gatherers are like Zen monks who attain well-being by choosing simplicity (1968); Michelle Rosaldo's expressions of sadness at the advent of development that had robbed Ilongot men of their head-hunting fun (1980); and Norberg-Hodge's assertions that Ladakhi people had little experience of ill-being and poverty until development came along, but that their ancient sense of "*joie de vivre*" has survived despite these modern sufferings (1991, 83). Even Chagnon, whose gleeful cataloguing of grotesque levels of violence is somewhat at odds with the biblical Eden, changed the title of his well-known book from *Yanamamö: The Fierce People* (1968) to *Yanamamö: The Last Days of Eden* (1992).

Such texts lack any plausible theory of comparative well-being. Similarly, the credibility of our discipline is not helped by the kind of uncritical romanticism exemplified by Bodley's entry (2004) in the online edition of *Encarta*, which assures readers that anthropologists don't believe in progress, that their relativist approach has allowed them to reveal "that every cultural group lives in a way that works well for many of its people," and that "anthropologists work from the assumption that a culture is effective and adaptive for the people who live in it ... [and that] a culture structures and gives meaning to the lives of its members and allows them to work and prosper." I trust that most anthropologists today would not pretend that all cultures are equally good, and would recognize in principle that some cultures, or institutions, beliefs, and practices, are better than others at allowing people to achieve well-being and to achieve meaningful lives.

Anthropologists do seem to be allowed to refer to the goodness of life in their book titles, but only on condition that the main text is actually about the badness of life. You can write a book about the *Anthropology of Welfare* that is almost entirely about ill-fare (Edgar and Russell 1998), or a book about *Mental Health* that is entirely about mental illness (Desjarlais et al. 1995), or a book about *Human Rights* that is entirely about human wrongs (Wilson 1997), or, hedging your bets, you can write a book on *Contentment and Suffering* purporting to cover both sides of the story, but then largely forget about the "contentment" part (Hollan and Wellenkamp 1994). Or you can just be an honest Tolstoyan, decide that extreme forms of ill-being and suffering are more interesting than well-being, and write about these without pausing to discuss what normal well-being might look like (Scheper-Hughes 1979, 1992; Kleinman and Good 1985; Kleinman et al. 1997).

Any discipline reluctant to study normality is going to have trouble studying well-being. It is this institutionalized incapacity that bedevils anthropology. It detracts from our relevance to the real world, and from our claims to scientific rigor and ethical standards. I am not arguing against the study of oddities as a route to understanding normality. But communities of scholars must be prepared to find themselves odd too. *The cold-shouldering of well-being by anthropologists is itself a bizarre feature of the culture of academic anthropology, one that begs to be analyzed.* How can a discipline that for over a century has promoted holistic analysis of the important dimensions of human life have had so little to say about well-being and its place in cultural debate and narratives about the meaning or purpose of life? How can so many of us have explored meanings, processes, and patternings of society and culture with scarcely a glance at the ways in which humans enjoy their lives, or at their views on well-being?

My argument is in part normative: to be relevant and respectable, anthropology must (not just could or should but *must*) do much more than it has so far done to theorize and collate our contributions to the understanding of well-being (and of its pursuit and moral valuation) in diverse cultural contexts. My argument is also intellectual and introspective: by analyzing the well-being deficit in anthropology, we can learn much about the history and culture of our discipline.

Background: A History of Interest in Well-Being

In the seventeenth to nineteenth centuries, the philosophers whose work eventually made modern social science possible wrote extensively about "happiness" and related concepts like "welfare" and "utility." Locke, Hobbes, Montesquieu, Condorcet, Marx, Comte, and Spencer were all explicitly interested in promoting better understanding of happiness, and also in its relevance to social analysis and social policy. Adam Smith and Malthus both affirmed that happiness is the ultimate human goal—although the replacement of happiness with wealth soon earned the discipline of economics the title of the "dismal science," and by the start of the twentieth century, Alfred Marshall (1902) was to declare that economics was no longer directly concerned with well-being but rather with material goods.

Durkheim's strong interest in happiness, life satisfaction, and health is evident in all of his key texts. The psychological traditions were also steeped in happiness theory until the silencing of happiness crept in. Wundt and Freud wrote extensively on the meaning of happiness and its role in social life. It is most prominent in the work of William James, whose *Varieties of Religious Experience* (1902) is almost obsessively focused on happiness—as the ultimate good, as a personality trait of religious entrepreneurs and hence as the source of religious faith, and as a moral objective for programs of mental self-control. Given the silencing of research into happiness that took place during the first half of the twentieth century, it wasn't until the 1960s that even a tiny minority of psychologists began to follow his advice and focus on positive emotion and its manipulability.

Well-being research throughout the twentieth century has largely been dominated by philosophers, theologians, moral crusaders, self-improvement gurus, and more recently by psychologists and economists. Even writings on cross-cultural perspectives on happiness are authored almost entirely by psychologists (e.g., see Diener and Suh 2000, whose nineteen authors are all psychologists). Reference books and introductory texts on anthropology (including even key textbooks on psychological anthropology such as Bock 1980, 1988; Harré and Parrott 1996 [1985]; Schwartz et al. 1992; and Segall et al. 1999) typically have no entries on happiness or well-being. Rapport and Overing's (2000) collection of sixty essays on "key concepts" in anthropology includes none on well-being, happiness, human flourishing, emotion, or quality of life. The subject index of the Routledge *Encyclopedia of Social and Cultural Anthropology* (Barnard and Spencer 1996) skips blithely from "habitus" to "harmonic regimes" and "haruspicy" without a thought for happiness, and from "warfare" to "Wenner-Gren Foundation" with no nod towards well-being. Unsurprisingly, therefore, Veenhoven's introduction to the *World Database of Happiness* (1997), which heralds a breakthrough in social science research on happiness as a complement to nonempirical philosophizing, and which argues in principle for cross-cultural comparative studies of happiness, recommends no anthropological readings on happiness.

Identifying and Interpreting the Deficit

Anthropology can contribute to the cross-cultural understanding of well-being, but not without theoretical debate, a foregrounding of well-being in the discipline, engagement with the research on well-being in other disciplines, and some careful consideration of why hitherto the anthropology of well-being has been so weak and inexplicit. In an earlier paper on the anthropology of happiness (Thin 2005), I argued that the cross-cultural study of happiness was inhibited in twentieth-century anthropology by four sets of factors, each of which is similarly applicable to the well-being deficit.

First, there has been a *relativist/adaptivist* bias against evaluation and evaluative comparison, and in favor of naïve romanticism about some non-Western cultures. In *Anthropology by Comparison,* Fox and Gingrich remind us of the sense of public responsibility that anthropologists felt in the 1920s and 1930s, part of which was to offer cultural comparisons that would be in the public interest. Since then, and particularly in the last two decades of the twentieth century, they argue, we have been neglecting cross-cultural comparison (2002, 1–3). Anthropologists have described situations and analyzed patterns without coming to explicit judgments about the good or bad quality of human experience. In anthropology and in cross-cultural or multicultural studies, relativism has acted as a strong deterrent against cross-cultural comparative moral judgments (for an excellent if pathological critique, see Edgerton 1992).

Second, the *pathological/clinical* bias has been more recently evident in the tendency to focus on suffering, ill-being, and adverse emotion. I have discussed this pervasive pathologism in the social sciences in my book *Social Progress and Sustainable Development* (2002). With well-being assumed as the default, ill-being attracts more commentary than well-being. Hollan and Wellenkamp tried to assess both "contentment" and "suffering" but focused on the latter, saying that for the Toraja they spoke and lived with, "happiness and contentment can best be defined as the occasional and fleeting absence of suffering and hardship" (1994, 28). Edgerton's critique of nonevaluative anthropology would have been better still if he had complemented his litany of maladaptive cultural practices with some portrayal of what an "adaptive" or "well" culture might look like.

Third, the *cognitivist/social constructionist* bias has steered anthropologists away from interpretation of emotions and experiences in social analysis. In part this bias arose in reaction to the excessive naturalism of biological determinists' and evolutionary psychologists' accounts of "basic emotions" and of their imputed influences on culture and social institutions. Rodney Needham's *Structure and Sentiment,* a structuralist manifesto against psychologism, epitomizes the cognitivist bias. He declared psychological interpretations of kinship systems to be "demonstrably wrong" (1962, vii–viii), and seemed oblivious to the simple point that no kind of account of kinship—whether it is descriptive, analytical, or normative—can reasonably be proposed without reference to the ways in which people emotionally experience kinship systems. Could this man be in some way related to the Rodney Needham who, just nineteen years later, was writing a scathing attack on anthropologists' failure to write about "inner states" as understood through "indigenous psychology" (Needham 1981, 56)? In this later work Needham exemplifies social constructionism, arguing reasonably enough that anthropologists' naïve belief in universal inner states had made them neglect psychology. Social constructionist anthropologists since then have produced a great deal of interesting work on emotion, but this has been marred both by its pathological bias and by its often clumsy attempts to portray social construction as a better alternative to evolutionary psychology rather than as complementary to it (for good critiques, see Lyon 1995; Reddy 1997, 2001).

Finally, the *antiutilitarian* and *antihedonistic* biases combine to restrict anthropological understanding of motives and pleasures. Starting with Frazer's preface to Malinowski's *Argonauts,* anthropologists have shunned so-called utilitarian motives and explanations, rejecting as ethnocentric Western economists' assumptions about rationality. In doing so, they have revealed their own ignorance of utilitarian philosophy. Malinowski claimed to be antiutilitarian, but was wrong to think that by describing Trobrianders as spending effort on yam cultivation that was "unnecessary … from a utilitarian point of view" (1978 [1922], 60), he was showing the irrelevance of modern economics to the interpretation of culture. Trobrianders *do,* as individuals, see such efforts as necessary for their well-being, as part of the meaning-making project of life. As Elvin Hatch has recently pointed out, Malinowski's own functionalist theory "assumed a universal standard of good" and "rested on … a version of utilitarian theory whereby the practical benefits of institutions served as a standard for making judgments" (1997, 373). And since "utility" for utilitarians ranges from pleasure (Bentham 1948 [1776]) to "worthy" happiness (Mill 1863), anthropologists wanting to engage with economists or moral philosophers would need to be able to make subtle distinctions among diverse kinds of pleasures and motives. Yet antihedonism has prevented us from taking pleasure seriously as an object of enquiry. When Plath proposed research on enjoyment in Japan, his colleagues "regarded the project as preposterously amusing" (1964, 8). In the happiness-embracing culture of the 1970s US, Freedman found many thousands of people willing to answer questionnaires on happiness, but his research assistant found ethnographic enquiry almost impossible as people would only discuss it frivolously in groups and were too embarrassed to discuss it at all in private (1978). Clark's chapter 9 in this book is an effort to redress the anthropological neglect of pleasure.

To summarize the implications of these biases:

- The *relativist/adaptivist* bias impedes our willingness to make evaluative comparisons of the performance of social institutions, cultural beliefs, and practices in generating well-being.

- The *pathological/clinical* bias limits our ability to say what makes people well or have a good life, as opposed to what makes them suffer and have a bad life.
- The *cognitivist/social constructionist* bias inhibits the discussion of feeling, impoverishing our descriptions and interpretations. When we do address feelings, the constructionist bias inhibits recognition of the intertwining of culture with genetic and biological factors in the generation of feeling.
- The *antiutilitarian/antihedonistic* bias prevents communication between anthropologists, moral philosophers, and economists on the meaning of utility and its relation to motives, and inhibits due recognition of the diversity of motives that are related to pleasure.

Three Kinds of Interest in Well-Being

"Well-being," like "happiness," may be too broad for analytical purposes. We must distinguish three kinds of reasons for studying well-being: to understand *feelings, evaluative meanings,* and *motives.*

- *Feelings:* Following the leads of the "anthropology of experience" and the "subjective well-being" movement, we must try to understand how people feel—about themselves in general, about relationships, institutions, processes, and events, and about the nonhuman environment. The idea of "feeling well" is the core meaning of "happiness." For psychologists, feeling well has two independent dimensions: having good feelings, and minimizing bad feelings. Many of our individual efforts and social policies are aimed more at minimizing suffering than at optimizing happiness.
- *Evaluative meanings:* Following the leads of moral philosophy and the "quality of life" and "social indicators" movements, we must try to understand how people make meaning in their lives by evaluating the quality of their own lives and those of other people, both in general and with reference to specific domains. This secondary meaning of "happiness" is better called "life satisfaction." As many famously miserable creative geniuses have shown, it is possible to "live a good life" (in that you and/or others evaluate your life positively) without much happiness. Many commentators on so-called collectivist societies have noted that people are less concerned with feeling good than they are in individualistic societies, because instead they emphasize living well in the prosocial sense (see Derné, chapter 6).

- *Motives:* Following the leads of various approaches to the study of motivation (in psychology, economics, and religious studies, as well as within anthropology itself), we need to explore the ultimate motives that end in themselves. Motives include not only the desire to feel good but also the desire to have a life that is "good" in the sense that it is meaningful and judged well by other people in accordance with social principles. Further, religious motives include the desire to be judged well by supernatural beings and to live well in an afterlife, and nature-lovers want to harmonize with the nonhuman environment.

Universals and Diversity in Well-Being

Building on these distinctions, I propose three assumptions about attitudes to well-being that have perhaps universal cross-cultural validity despite occasional skeptical or countercultural philosophies:

- In all cultures, most people most of the time want to feel good and want to make the other people with whom they empathize feel good. Concepts of well-feeling play central roles in individual and collective motives.
- All cultures distinguish "feeling well" from "living a good life," and base much of their moral debate and existential meaning-making on this distinction.
- All core moral codes (despite rhetorical countermoralities) endorse the idea that it is better in principle (i.e., in the absence of exceptional strategic reasons such as punishments) to try to help other people to feel well and to live a good life than to try to make other people feel bad and live a bad life.

In response to academic neglect, such statements assert the universality of popular interest in well-being and remind us that well-being matters in diverse ways that aren't just about individuals feeling well. Far from pushing well-being into the background domain of uninteresting truism, these claims about universals pave the way for careful analysis of how approaches to well-being differ among individuals and according to cultural context.

The diversity of well-being concepts and motives are worth exploring more fully than has been done so far. We must recognize that individuals, cultures, and specific cultural contexts vary in their degree of emphasis on hedonism (valuing good feeling, wanting to feel good, and by extension wanting to make others feel good) versus evaluative meaning (valuing lives that are rich in meaning). In some philosophies, happiness is defined as just one among several life purposes—ranking alongside rather than above others such as virtue, religious merit, and knowledge. We may all want to feel good, but we vary greatly in the degree of deferment that we are willing to accept. Some individuals and cultures may see lifelong daily happiness as the desired norm. Others put much more emphasis on working, suffering, and deferring pleasures now in order to achieve happiness later in life or in an afterlife.

Discussions about altruism can similarly be helped by exploring unities and diversities in attitudes to well-being. People vary in the extent to which they see their well-being as dependent on other peoples' well-being, or on their contributions to others' well-being. The concept of altruism itself can refer either to making other people feel good, or to helping them lead worthy lives. Furthermore, there are diverse views on how to achieve well-being, and great variation in people's ability to imagine and respect other people's and other cultures' alternative routes to well-being.

Norms for the display of well-being are also highly variable. Attitudes or principles concerning the display of happiness vary in terms of whether it is good to display it in general, and in terms of whether happiness display is more or less appropriate for young or old people, men or women. Situations vary too (is it good or bad form to be happy at weddings or at funerals?) as do relational contexts (is it good or bad form to be cheerful and smiling in the company of a superior?). So too with the meaningfulness or worthiness of lives: this may be a matter for public display or something to be kept strictly private.

Axes of Semantic Distinction

To understand how "well-being" is used, we must identify the axes along which differentiations of meaning are made. The list below suggests some lines of enquiry that would help us to identify how the terms are used.

Positive versus Neutral

Well-being sounds positive, but can be used in a neutral sense as in common neutral uses of height or breadth or health. Ironically, this neutral usage allows well-being to be used as a heading for texts on ill-being. It is also theoretically possible to distinguish *value-laden* or *normative* versus *value-free* uses of "well-being": for most people the term implies values and value judgments, but it is possible to describe well-being concepts without being judgmental.

Residualist versus Constructive Approaches

The World Health Organization has made famous the idea that health is more than the absence of illness, and that well-being is more than just the absence of ill-being. Yet most institutions and texts relating to health and well-being still treat these concepts in a residualist way as the (hypothetical) absence of avoidable suffering or impairment. Most activity and policy under the health and well-being rubrics is about ridding people of illness and avoidable suffering. The need for constructive rather than residualist approaches arises in part because well-being requires not just an escape from harm but a set of balances between undesirable extremes. The UN buzz-phrase of progress as the "expansion of choice" arose from recognition that poor people have restricted choice, but as a slogan for progress it is inept, since people need enough choice to pursue well-being but not so much that they are confused all the time. Nor are *security* or *peace* equivalent to social goods if they are too complete: individually and collectively we depend for our happiness on some amount of indeterminacy and disturbance in our lives, so the removal of insecurity and conflict are not in themselves viable strategies for well-being.

Short-term versus Long-term Orientation

Pleasure and *joy* tend to refer to relatively short-term or momentary well-being, whereas *life satisfaction, happiness,* and *fulfillment* tend to refer to long-term orientation. Much of the debate about the morality of hedonism turns on the semantics of pleasure, and specifically on whether or not it means mainly private, short-term, and bodily pleasure or more prosocial, lasting, and mental or "higher" pleasures.

This-worldly versus Other-worldly Orientation

Most people worldwide anticipate an afterlife. Many also aspire to and apparently enjoy experiences or states of being called, for example, "ecstasy" or "bliss" that are "otherworldly" in that they happen outside normal consciousness. The Buddhist concept of nirvana shares some of the semantic meanings of well-being and happiness, but is also distinctive to the extent that it emphasizes detachment from normal sources of both well-being and suffering.

Experiential versus Conceptual or Evaluative Orientation

Accounts of well-being can be about people's actual *experiences,* or about their *conceptualizations* of their experiences. Too many reports from surveys eliciting information about self-reported happiness forget this crucial distinction, and slip too easily from factual assertions about self-reports to speculative assertions about how happy people are. Mathews in chapter 8 recommends that anthropologists focus mainly on concepts rather than experiences, since the latter are too elusive for study. A different but closely related distinction is between *emotional* and *cognitive* meanings—between *feeling* well and *thinking* we are well.

Subjective versus Objective Well-Being

Subjective well-being means happiness in the sense of feeling good. Hollan in chapter 10 sees individual subjective experience as the core meaning of well-being. But both of these terms may be extended to include assessments of well-being, which, although still focused on individuals' experience, are also objective to the extent that they treat the experiencer (who may be the self doing the appraising) as an object to be studied. When social psychologists ask people questions like "Taking all things as a whole, how well would you say your life is going?" they are assessing life satisfaction, but they often call this "subjective well-being." Actually these are *objective* assessments (by researchers) of *objective* assessments (by informants) of their own *subjective* feelings.

Aggregative versus Integrated Assessment

Jeremy Bentham's utilitarian ideal of a "felicific calculus," never implemented despite his detailed lists, is the defining example of an aggregative approach to well-being. He saw happiness as the sum of pleasures minus pains. Most people more sensibly recognize that the process of assessing well-being, while it may involve some degree of mental addition and subtraction, is more importantly a process of *meaning-making,* interpreting the quality of life in an integrated way.

Domain-specific versus Holistic/Inclusive Assessment

Inclusive (or "global") assessments of well-being are problematic because of noncomparabilities between different domains of experience. Some researchers find it more meaningful to assess well-being in specific domains. The kind of happiness we seek or expect at work might be seen as utterly different from the kinds of happiness we associate with family life or leisure activities or religion. Whereas terms like *flourishing* and *happiness* are multidomain inclusive terms, *flow* can be either inclusive or can refer to good feelings that derive from a very specific activity, and *fun* refers to the moods or feelings deriving from a fairly restrictive set of activities belonging in the leisure domain.

Physiological versus Metaphysical Assessment

Well-being is commonly used restrictively as a fashionable synonym for health. In English, the core meaning of *well* is understood as referring to the body, so that "feeling well" in the health sense can be distinguished from "feeling good" in the more holistic sense, including mental well-being. For this reason, anthropologists wanting to make more inclusive analysis of well-being might sensibly choose a more obviously inclusive term like *flourishing,* or complement attention to well-being with attention to *happiness,* which clearly has metaphysical meanings beyond health alone.

Egocentric versus Sociocentric Assessment

Most discussion of well-being focuses primarily on individuals, and only secondarily on the social systems and relations that facilitate or inhibit individual well-being. Arguably, though, well-being and related concepts can be applied to aggregates of people. Nations or cultures are sometimes described as "well" or "sick," and social occasions can be "happy" or "sad." Not everyone readily understands the idea of assessing well-being from an egocentric point of view. The stereotypical North American/European view of happiness as a personal pursuit has been said to be anathema to people from collectivist societies who assess well-being in sociocentric ways. This is discussed at length by Derné in chapter 6 and by Heil in chapter 4.

Arousal versus Calm

Is the quality of a person's life best evaluated according to its excitement or according to its quietude? This kind of question has long exercised philosophers, and it occasionally surfaces in anthropology—explicitly in Hollan and Wellenkamp's discussion of Toraja views on contentment as the fleeting absence of suffering (1994, 28), and implicitly in Rosaldo's sadness at the demise of head-hunting that had allowed men to enjoy a high-contrast life of indulgence in peaks of high-energy rage followed by periods of calm (1980). "Happiness" poses analytic problems because it covers both extremes of the arousal-calm continuum, serving as a synonym for both exuberant joy and quiet contentment.

Where Would Anthropologies of Well-Being Fit In?

There are a number of key areas of anthropological study that simply *must* make well-being central to their enquiries. Research and writing on morality, value, development, human rights, poverty, health, and mental health all fall into this category. All offer promising opportunities for engagements with happiness studies, moral philosophy, and the social indicators movement. All these areas of anthropological enquiry, to varying degrees, have fallen short of adequate engagement with discussions of well-being.

The well-being deficit is most conspicuous in the anthropologies of morality and value, which have been rightly declared by their exponents to be strikingly weak areas of anthropology (Edel and Edel 1959; Overing 1985; Howell 1997; Laidlaw 2001; Graeber 2002). Laidlaw has argued, reasonably, that "there cannot be ... [an] anthropology of ethics without ... an ethnographic and theoretical interest ... in freedom" (2001, 311). But like most of the anthropologists writing about ethics, Laidlaw misses the most fundamental weakness, namely the lack of any theorizing of well-being in both anthropological ethics and in the anthropology of ethics. We need to ask the question: "Freedom to do what?" We could then argue that there cannot be an anthropology of ethics or of freedom without developing an anthropology of the ultimate goods that we might be free to choose. You cannot plausibly discuss good behavior without discussing people's views and rationales concerning good feelings and good lives.

So while ethnographies and cross-cultural analyses of value systems and moralities have provided helpful insights for the study of well-being, they have not themselves been evaluative in relation to a set of well-being criteria. Ethnography is not entirely nonevaluative. Many anthropologists have written passionate accounts of avoidable suffering, violence, and repression, telling of children denied the opportunity to play, adolescents and circumcised women denied sexual enjoyment, commoners denied livelihoods and dignity, and women battered or murdered by husbands and kin. But without a basis in some comparative account of universals and diversities in well-being concepts and experiences, such moral critiques are on shaky ground even when they resonate with the "gut feelings" of most readers. This comment applies particularly well to Raoul Naroll, whose ambitious and idiosyncratic work *The Moral Order* (1983) is a rare attempt at systematic cross-cultural comparison of well-being and morality. Seeking to demonstrate that "moralnets" (dense networks of good social connections) are the key to happiness worldwide, Naroll approached this challenge without a clear concept or theory or ethnography of well-being, and by measuring not well-being but a list of "social ills."

Similarly, it is embarrassing for the discipline to have professional codes of ethics (e.g., ASA 1999; AAA 1998) that pontificate on the good behavior of anthropologists, and on their responsibilities towards the well-being of the people they study and of humanity in general, with no reference to any theories or empirical studies of well-being or happiness. It is similarly awkward that collections of secondary texts discussing anthropological ethics (Fluehr-Lobban 2002 [1991]; Caplan 2003; Meskell and Pels 2005) show virtually no interest in well-being.

In clinical anthropologies of development, human rights, poverty, health, and mental health, anthropologists are indeed concerned with well-being, but in a residualist way. The problem here is largely with the emphasis on pathology that has prevented these anthropologists from distinguishing the avoidance of ill-being from the promotion of well-being. Anthropologists involved in applied work in these domains have focused mainly on the avoidance and relief of harm and suffering, downplaying the different challenges of conceptualizing, assessing, and promoting well-being. Development anthropologists focus on poverty and/or on the harm done by bad development policies and projects. Human rights anthropologists, like human rights theorists and activists more generally, focus almost exclusively on human wrongs, as I have mentioned. Arguably the most striking and important instance of the pathological bias is the *World Mental Health* report (Desjarlais et al. 1995). This was perhaps anthropology's biggest opportunity to make a global impact on the cross-cultural understanding of well-being. It made useful contributions to the appreciation of the diverse concepts, causes, and treatments of mental illness, but had little to say about mental health. After acknowledging that "mental health is not simply the absence of detectable mental disease but a state of well-being" (1996, 7), the authors forgot about well-being altogether.

Health ethnographies use the term *well-being* from time to time, but largely without exploring its meanings. Wallman and her coauthors' book *Kampala Women Getting By: Wellbeing in the Time of AIDS* is an interesting ethnography, but lacks any substantial analytical contributions to the understanding of well-being. Well-being is mainly understood here as a slight broadening of the concept of health, not as a focus for discussion of ultimate human values or the rich diversity of valued experiences. Still less in evidence is any overall ethical conclusion about quality of life. Some effort was made to elicit women's views on "feeling good," but the book has little to say about how they actually feel about life in general, and concludes lamely that "inevitably questions of feeling are subject to interpretation and not suited to empirical survey" (Wallman et al. 1996, 108–10), thereby implicitly condemning as worthless all social psychologists' efforts to measure happiness, but not offering anything else in their place.

In the third of three volumes on "social suffering," Das et al. (2001) give an unfulfilled introductory promise that the essays are about the "reimagination of well-being" and about people remaking their lives after severe social traumas. Interpreting such accounts can offer important insights based on the extraordinary fact that people continue to remain alive and human at all, let alone achieve well-being, following such obscene shocks and suffering. Yet the essays don't address well-being as an achievement or as an aspiration, nor do they discuss the relevance of these extreme scenarios to other kinds of human situations. Similarly, Kleinman's other contributions to the anthropology of mental illness and suffering could have been more instructive if they had included cultural accounts of well-being. Scheper-Hughes's *Saints, Scholars, and Schizophrenics* (1979), a popular classic on mental illness, unhappiness, "demoralization," and "cultural disintegration," offers 240 pages of unmitigated misery without pausing to consider who, in rural western Ireland in the 1970s, was mentally well, or what their aspirations and concepts of well-being were.

Another set of problems in these clinical domains arises from a focus on interim processes rather than ultimate values and outcomes. Edgar and Russell's *The Anthropology of Welfare* (1998) promises in its promotional blurb to "provide an overview of what anthropology has to offer welfare studies and vice-versa." Yet by using "welfare" in the ethnocentric and narrow sense of European state policies for addressing particular kinds of unmet need and suffering, it forgets the cross-cultural approach altogether. The book also ignores well-being, focusing instead on dependency, community support, and service provision to disadvantaged people. Worthy though such accounts may be, it is baffling that authors didn't think to base their (usually implicit) advocacy for improved welfare services on any kind of theory of well-being and its causes, and that they did not think a cross-cultural perspective on well-being and on welfare services might have helped. By contrast, the social psychologist Ruut Veenhoven (2000) did systematically analyze well-being and welfare services across forty nations from 1980 to

1990: his findings show a controversially awkward lack of correlation between so-called welfare investments and well-being outcome measures. Since part of the controversy turns on how to define well-being across such diverse contexts, it is easy to see how some detailed ethnographic data and analysis on well-being could helpfully insert itself into policy debate.

Two other major recent collections of well-being studies conducted mainly by sociologists—Bradshaw's review of *The Well-being of Children in the UK* (2002) and Hermalin's four-country study of *The Well-Being of the Elderly in Asia* (2002)—might perhaps have been greatly enriched through the contributions from anthropologists' qualitative ethnographies and holistic analysis. But neither anthropologists nor even the theme of well-being itself got invited to the party. Look beyond the cover or the title of most "well-being" texts and you will find little about well-being. Just as the majority of "mental health" texts are actually about mental illness, so "well-being" is typically used as a euphemism for discussions of poverty, ill-health, and suffering. To team up effectively with other social scientists in order to enrich understanding of well-being, anthropologists will have to fight not only for recognition of the value of cross-cultural and ethnographic approaches, but also for recognition of well-being in the positive, constructive sense that the term implies.

In addition to these areas where explicit interest in well-being is essential, there are many other strands of anthropological enquiry that could clearly benefit from insertion of well-being themes. These are indicated in Table 1.1.

Conclusion

People everywhere show concern for the well-being of people they encounter and care about. To be humane, indeed to be authentically anthropological, anthropologists must show that they share this concern. Conventions for greetings show some of the diversity of this concern. When I first visited India, I was struck by two kinds of greetings uttered in Indian English. People would often ask me: "Have you taken your meals?" or "Your parents, they are there?" Both enquired about my well-being, but quite differently from the "How are you?" question I had been brought up with. The "meals" question shows a strong cultural emphasis on food as an idiom of social relations. If someone is hungry, it is a potential constraint on the relationship you may have with them: either you must be polite and feed them, or avoid them. Among poorer

Table 1.1 Potential Engagements between Anthropology and Well-Being Studies

1. Essential engagements

Anthropology of...	Rationale for engagement
Morality, value, altruism, philanthropy, and religion	Serious discussion of morality is not possible without reference to theories of the good, or what it means for a human life to go well. The anthropology of religion offers important insights into the collective generation of well-being, and into concepts of well-being in utopian visions and beliefs about after-life rewards.
Development, human rights, and progress	Activities and policies aimed at promoting "goods" and/or eliminating "bads" must be based in analysis of how ultimate goods are defined.
Ill-being, poverty, suffering, and harm	While ill-being is not just the converse of well-being, the two concepts are closely related and in part mutually constituted, so no analysis of ill-being is adequate without theorizing of well-being.
Health, mental health	These two concepts between them account for a major part of what "well-being" means. Yet most anthropological writing under these rubrics actually belongs under the "ill-being" rubric, and its inadequacy stems from a generalized failure to consider what people consider health or mental health to be.

2. Desirable engagements

Anthropology of ...	Rationale for engagement
Politics	The "who gets what, when, where, and why" questions beg for analysis of the different well-being outcomes for different categories of people under different kinds of political regimes and processes. Political anthropologists could also discuss what utilitarian policies and their outcomes might look like, and how they might be interpreted, in different cultural contexts.
Violence and peacemaking	It is time to overcome the pathological bias and explore the cross-cultural understanding of the peace, security, and excitement components in well-being.
Consumption	Consumption theorists could go beyond their analysis of symbolic meanings of goods, displays, and exchanges, and link the analysis of the desire for goods with the analysis of well-being concepts and aspirations.
Work	Studies of work are inadequate if they do not represent the affective and meaningful dimensions of the quality of working life.
Leisure, play, sport	Given their close association with pleasure and fun, leisure activities are essential components in all people's conceptions of the good life.

people, at least in the past, the ever-present threat of hunger would no doubt lead to a close equation between well-being and food. The question about the "thereness" of my parents is rather more complex, seeking assurance of my basic social connectedness but perhaps also revealing a deeper concern with the existential dimension of well-being.

Two anthropological articles on well-being have recently discussed this theme. Charlton's speculative article on evolution and "the meaning of life" (2002) argues that humanity evolved as a species that felt (as hunter-gatherers) both "happy" and "at home in the world," and that feelings of division and alienation are by-products of cultural change since the development of agriculture. In this account, concern with well-being would have been unnecessary for most of humanity's existence as hunter-gatherers. Agriculturalists would later have developed concern for well-being as part of their worries about the food supply and about the social placements through which production, distribution, and consumption of food is organized. This latter is well illustrated in Beverly and Whittemore's account of how rural Mandinka people in Senegal enquire about well-being. Adult greetings are not "How are you?" "I am well" but "Where is your mother?" "She is there." Such exchanges "express the ideal state of well-being. ... To be 'there' where one is supposed to be, is to be fine and at home in the Mandinka world" (1993, 270). These two items, like the ethnographies in this collection, well exemplify the rich interpretive possibilities of the anthropology of well-being.

This chapter has identified the inadequate attention to well-being in most anthropological work so far, and explored the causes of that inadequacy and the damage it does to the discipline. Anthropological engagement with the fundamentals of moral debate has been embarrassingly weak, and to set that right we must make the comparative analytical and empirical study of well-being central to our concerns. Without such attention, we cannot expect to offer adequate descriptions of human experience or human nature. By developing an anthropology of well-being, we will greatly improve our ability to offer culturally sophisticated contributions towards making the world a better place for people to live in.

References

American Anthropological Association [AAA]. 1998. *Code of Ethics of the American Anthropological Association.* http://www.aaanet.org/committees/ethics/ethcode.htm. Accessed 23 April 2006.

Association of Social Anthropologists [ASA]. 1999. *Ethical guidelines*. http://www .theasa.org/ethics.htm. Accessed 23 April 2006.
Barnard, Alan and Jonathan Spencer, eds. 1996. *Encyclopedia of Social and Cultural Anthropology*. London: Routledge.
Bentham, Jeremy. 1948 [1776]. *Introduction to the Principles of Morals and Legislation*. Oxford: Blackwell.
Beverly, Elizabeth and Robert D. Whittemore. 1993. "Mandinka Children and the Geography of Well-being." *Ethos* 21 (3): 235–72.
Bock, Philip K. 1980/1988. *Rethinking Psychological Anthropology. Continuity and Change in the Study of Human Action*. New York: W.H. Freeman and Co.
Bodley, John H. 2004. "Anthropology." *Encarta (Microsoft Online Encyclopedia)* http://encarta.msn.com/text_761559816__57/Anthropology.html. Accessed 23 April 2006.
Bradshaw, Jonathan, ed. 2002. *The Well-being of Children in the UK*. London: Save the Children.
Caplan, Pat, ed. 2003. *Ethics of Anthropology: Debates and Dilemmas*. London: Routledge.
Chagnon, Napoleon. 1968. *Yanamamö: The Fierce People*. New York: Holt, Rinehart and Winston.
———. 1992. *Yanamamö: The Last Days of Eden*. New York: Holt, Rinehart and Winston.
Charlton, Bruce G. 2002. "What is the Meaning of Life? Animism, Generalised Anthropomorphism and Social Intelligence." http://www.hedweb.com/ bgcharlton/meaning-of life.html. Accessed 23 April 2006.
Das, Veena, Arthur Kleinman, Margaret Lock, Mamphela Ramphele, and Pamela Reynolds, eds. 2001. *Remaking a World: Violence, Social Suffering, and Recovery*. Berkeley: University of California Press.
Desjarlais, Robert, Leon Eisenberg, Byron Good, and Arthur Kleinman, eds. 1995. *World Mental Health: Problems and Priorities in Low-Income Countries*. New York, Oxford University Press.
Diener, Ed and Carol Diener. 1996. "Most People are Happy." *Psychological Science* 7 (3): 1811–85.
Diener, Ed and Eunkook M. Suh, eds. 2000. *Culture and Subjective Well-Being*. Cambridge, MA: MIT Press.
Edel, May and Abraham Edel. 1959. *Anthropology and Ethics*. Springfield, IL: Charles Thomas.
Edgar, Iain and Andrew Russell, eds. 1998. *The Anthropology of Welfare*. London: Routledge.
Edgerton, Robert. 1992. *Sick Societies: Challenging the Myth of Primitive Harmony*. New York: Free Press.
Eriksen, Thomas Hylland. 1995. *Small Places, Large Issues: An Introduction to Social and Cultural Anthropology*. London: Pluto Press.
Fox, Richard D. and Andre Gingrich, eds. 2002. *Anthropology by Comparison*. London: Routledge.
Fluehr-Lobban, Carolyn, ed. 2002 [1991]. *Ethics and the Profession of Anthropology: Dialogue for Ethically Conscious Practice*. Philadelphia: University of Pennsylvania Press / AltaMira Press.
Freedman, Jonathan L. 1978. *Happy People*. New York: Harcourt Brace.

Graeber, David. 2002. *Towards an Anthropological Theory of Value: The False Coin of Our Own Dreams.* London: Palgrave.

Harré, Rom and W. Gerrod Parrott. 1996 [1985]. *The Emotions: Social, Cultural and Biological Dimensions.* London: Sage.

Hatch, Elvin. 1997. "The Good Side of Relativism." *Journal of Anthropological Research* 53 (3): 371–82.

Hermalin, Albert I. 2002. *The Well-Being of the Elderly in Asia: A Four-Country Comparative Study.* Ann Arbor: University of Michigan Press.

Hollan, Douglas W. and Jane C. Wellenkamp. 1994. *Contentment and Suffering: Culture and Experience in Toraja.* New York: Columbia University Press.

Howell, Signe, ed. 1997. *The Ethnography of Moralities.* London: Routledge.

James, William. 1902. *The Varieties of Religious Experience.* London: Longmans.

Kleinman, Arthur and Byron Good, eds. 1985. *Culture and Depression.* Berkeley: University of California Press.

Kleinman, Arthur, Veena Das and Margaret Lock, eds. 1997. *Social Suffering.* Berkeley: University of California Press.

Laidlaw, James. 2001. "For an Anthropology of Ethics and Freedom." *Journal of the Royal Anthropological Institute* 8: 311–332.

Lévi-Strauss, Claude. 1973 [1955]. *Tristes Tropiques.* Trans. John and Doreen Weightman. New York: Washington Square Press.

Lyon, Margot. 1995. "Missing Emotion: The Limitations of Cultural Constructionism in the Study of Emotion." *Cultural Anthropology* 10 (2): 244–63.

Malinowski, Bronislaw. 1978 [1922]. *Argonauts of the Western Pacific.* London: Routledge.

Marshall, Alfred. 1902. "Economic Teaching at the Universities in Relation to Public Wellbeing." Paper presented to the Committee on Social Education, Charity Organisation Society, London. Summarized in *Economic Journal* 13 (49): 155.

Marshall, Lorna. 1959. *The Harmless People.* London: Secker and Warburg.

Meskell, Lynn and Peter Pels. 2005. *Embedding Ethics: Shifting Boundaries of the Anthropological Profession.* Oxford: Berg.

Mill, John Stuart. 1863. *Utilitarianism.* http://www.constitution.org/jsm/utilitarianism.txt. Accessed 23 April 2006.

Naroll, Raoul. 1983. *The Moral Order: An Introduction.* Beverly Hills: Sage.

Needham, Rodney. 1962. *Structure and Sentiment.* Chicago: University of Chicago Press.

———. 1981. *Circumstantial Deliveries.* Berkeley: University of California Press.

Norberg-Hodge, Helena. 1991. *Ancient Futures: Learning from Ladakh.* London: Rider.

Overing, Joanna. 1985. *Reason and Morality.* London: Tavistock.

Plath, David. 1964. *The After Hours: Modern Japan and the Search for Enjoyment.* Berkeley: University of California Press.

Rapport, Nigel and Joanna Overing. 2000. *Social and Cultural Anthropology: The Key Concepts.* London: Routledge.

Reddy, William M. 1997. "Against Constructionism: The Historical Ethnography of Emotions." *Current Anthropology* 38 (3): 327–51.

———. 2001. *The Navigation of Feeling: A Framework for the History of Emotions.* Cambridge: Cambridge University Press.

Rosaldo, Michelle Z. 1980. *Knowledge and Passion: Ilongot Notions of Self and Social Life.* Cambridge: Cambridge University Press.

Sahlins, Marshall D. 1968. "Notes on the Original Affluent Society." In *Man the Hunter,* ed. Richard B. Lee and Irven DeVore, 858–59. Chicago: Aldine.

Scheper-Hughes, Nancy. 1979. *Saints, Scholars, and Schizophrenics: Mental Illness in Rural Ireland.* Berkeley: University of California Press.

————. 1992. *Death Without Weeping.* Berkeley: University of California Press.

Schwartz, Theodore, Geoffrey M. White, and Catherine A. Lutz, eds. 1992. *New Directions in Psychological Anthropology.* Cambridge: Cambridge University Press.

Segall, Marshall H., Pierre R. Dasen, John W. Berry, and Ype H. Poortinga, eds. 1999. *Human Behavior in Global Perspective: An Introduction to Cross Cultural Psychology.* 2nd ed. Boston: Allyn & Bacon/Longman.

Thin, Neil. 2002. *Social Progress and Sustainable Development.* London: ITDG Publications.

————. 2005. "Happiness and the Sad Topics of Anthropology." University of Bath: Wellbeing in Developing Countries Working Paper No. 10. http://www.welldev.org.uk/research/workingpaperpdf/wed10.pdf. Accessed 23 April 2006.

Turnbull, Colin M. 1961. *The Forest People.* London: Chatto & Windus.

Veenhoven, Ruut. 1997. "World Database of Happiness: Correlational Findings, Introductory Text." http://www.eur.nl/fsw/research/happiness/hap_cor/introtxt1.rtf. Accessed 4 April 2003.

————. 2000. "Well-being in the Welfare State: Level Not Higher, Distribution Not More Equitable." *Journal of Comparative Policy Analysis* 2: 911–25.

Wallman, Sandra et al. 1996. *Kampala Women Getting By: Wellbeing in the Time of AIDS.* London: James Currey.

Wilson, Richard A., ed. 1997. *Human Rights, Culture and Context: Anthropological Perspectives.* London: Pluto Press.

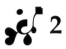 2

Is a Measure of Cultural Well-Being Possible or Desirable?

Benjamin Nick Colby

Any study of well-being, however characterized (cultural, sociocultural, psychocultural, social) must consider both the level and objective of analysis. At the very simplest, one can measure a psychological state, a state of subjective well-being or happiness with a five-item questionnaire about how satisfied respondents are with their lives (Diener and Suh 2000). One can go further by asking people what makes them happy, or how they define a successful life. These answers can be ranged along different levels of generality. A more detailed ethnography of people's goals, values, and attitudes will produce a large amount of data that then must be processed ethnographically. However, aside from ethnography-based, or primary-data approaches, there is a different, theory-based approach that has rarely been attempted by anthropologists in the study of cultural well-being. In this chapter, following a discussion of the nature and history of the anthropological study of well-being, I discuss the foundations of one such theory. But let me begin with the problem of culture.

The Problem of Culture and Cultural Relativism

A major reason why anthropologists have shied away from investigation into well-being, and a major hurdle that theory-based approaches to well-being have to surmount, is the problem of cultural relativism. This problem is illustrated by what I call Freud's impasse. In his *Civilizations and its Discontents,* Freud speculated that it would be quite possible for an entire culture or civilization to be psychologically sick (he said neurotic) just as an individual might be (1961 [1930], 102). However, Freud went on to point out a difference between the diagnosis of a culture and that of a single person. Individuals can be judged to be sick on the basis of how they differ from the norm. But who is to say what the norm for a culture or an entire civilization might be? There is no way, Freud argued, to determine norms for such an entity (1961 [1930], 103).

I am convinced that Freud was wrong, in that he based his argument on an inadequate theory of culture. He was using the conventional view of his day—one that happens to be, in its essentials, the same notion of culture used by anthropologists and the general public even now. This is the notion of culture as superorganic, as an autonomous entity that transcends individual human beings. This was applied to everything from a civilization to a band or tribal society. Most subjects of ethnography in the first half of the twentieth century lived in relatively small groups, localized in some particular geography. With the shift in compass from a broader civilization to a narrower island view, the word *culture* was often used in the plural or used as a count noun rather than a mass noun, that is, a specific set of patterns in some coherent configuration rather than a broader, less bounded view of culture as a mass, like water or sand. In either case, however, culture was seen as above and beyond biology and hence "superorganic." This attached to culture a sense of spurious natural history. Just as people classified butterflies or other orders of animals, so also might one distinguish and classify different cultures by their often strange or colorful characteristics.

This superorganic notion, and its numerous variations as a spurious natural history unit, was handed down from Boas through Kroeber, Herskovits, Benedict, and other anthropologists among Boas' students in the first half of the twentieth century. That same notion, usually in the narrower island or tribal variant, is still with us. As long as we keep to this view of culture as a count noun, as something over and above the biology of individuals, ethnographic studies of cultural well-being are not likely to provide a cumulative basis others can build upon with any success.

The major reason for Freud's impasse in determining the normality of culture was the relativism usually associated with this idea of culture, rendering comparison impossible: each bounded culture, this view holds, has its own unique patterns and ethos that cannot be judged vis-à-vis other cultures. But there are other problems closely tied up with cultural relativism. The locality of culture is a major one. First of all there is the matter of geographical locality. But then there is also physiological (does culture reside in our heads?) or even metaphysical locality. Before thinking about just where culture resides (and the question does seem relevant if we use culture as a count noun) we have to consider just what culture is, an ontological question.

Early on, anthropologists studied personality as separate from culture. Those studies were classified as "culture and personality." Later, especially with the rise of cognitive anthropology and the interest in language as part of culture, there were cracks in the superorganic idea. Does culture reside in people's heads, or is it outside, an entity, however ethereal, to which people belong? Is it a mere abstraction invented by anthropologists? Regardless of one's answer to these questions, culture was still seen as disjunctive with biology. Culture remained a nebulous concept, sometimes as patterned but with little systemic specification. Without a biological connection, there was little accounting for the emotional sources of motivation. There was thus no source of dynamics, no explanation of culture change; hence, the key process of culture transmission was given little attention in the detail needed.

This static, unworkable conventional view of culture carries over to other matters that create exclusionary contrasts: theory versus description, questionnaires versus interviewing, testing versus thick description, single cultural unit description versus cross-cultural comparison. An anthropology of the future will have to set aside these either-or characterizations. In the years ahead, anthropologists will likely find themselves active on both sides of such contrasts in their work.

Anthropology will require many perspectives, methods, and interdisciplinary contacts to meet the unprecedented challenges that lie in our future. Fresh, new approaches will be needed. Yet within the discipline it is rare to find answers to this call. Up until now, urgency for anthropological research has been for people whose culture is rapidly changing or disappearing, as, for example, studies supported by the Anthropologists' Fund for Urgent Anthropological Research. In the future, however, problems may beset the world as a whole, including some of the richest countries of the West, where many anthropologists themselves live, and where large-scale natural disasters and socioeconomic disruptions can negatively impact culture change in the direction of markedly lower levels of cultural well-being. The studies in this book, directed as they are to different approaches and ideas relating to well-being, represent a beginning in the answer to this call.

Now, under threat of political changes inimical to democracy, environmental changes due to technological culture, and the threat of pandemics, we are questioning who we are, what kind of society we live in, and, in the midst of so many changes ahead, both natural and technological, what kinds of lives we want to lead and what kinds of lives our fellow humans will have elsewhere on the planet in what is likely to be a very different future. Suddenly, cultural relativism seems to be weakening as a predominant feature of the anthropological landscape; even more pervasively, it is weakening in everyday speech.

The word *culture* has increasingly taken on an evaluational component in the public realm, in direct contradiction to a neutral relativistic view of particular "cultures" many anthropologists have tended to hold. These days we read about "the predatory culture of Enron," or "the culture of newsrooms" (described negatively). The increased occurrence of the term *culture* among the politically concerned public points to a rising focus on the quality of culture and the life that can be lived in today's social environments. Much of the public in the United States doesn't want to be relativistic about the dishonest executives at Enron, or take a relativistic stance with regard to the culture of torture in the military and in covert agencies, or the dismantling of cultural institutions set up to protect and support members of a society when they find themselves in difficulty.

Is this evaluating usage of the word *culture* to remain simply a vernacular usage, or do we need a parallel development in anthropology itself? The studies of well-being reported in this book show that there is a need, a response to the times, by anthropologists. The difficulty in such an enterprise, however, lies in two formidable problems: the relativity question, responsible for Freud's impasse; and the social complexity question, where the enormous variety of sociocultural elements characteristic of modern societies today poses real problems and calls for a more precise, scientifically useful theory of culture.

Often questions about cultural well-being or pathology come down to particular practices, beliefs, or attitudes on the part of one segment of the population toward another. This can become enormously complex when ideas about cultural relativity and multiculturalism conflict with ideas about well-being. In Holland, for example, 5.5 percent of the Dutch population is Muslim, yet half the women in battered women's shelters are Muslim and there are many more suicides among Muslim women than non-Muslim ones. There are similar statistics elsewhere in Europe. Honor killings of Muslim girls for dating non-Muslims have occurred, and female genital mutilation starting at six years of age is practiced among a subset of Muslim immigrants. Many other Muslim differences exist that create a radical divergence from the norm in Dutch society. Dutch commitment to cultural relativism as a form of tolerance may thus have had an adverse effect. It encouraged the continuance of feminine apartheid among Muslims and in so doing has resulted in major disruptions in the larger society in Holland. When a Muslim murdered an activist opposed to Muslim customs, the resulting reactions among the far right in Holland led to burning mosques and Islamic schools. The more liberal Dutch element finds itself divided over what to do. Through a hands-off tolerance, the Dutch have contributed to, rather than ameliorated, the repression of Islamic women immigrants in Holland.

Where does that leave the ethnographer? Ideally ethnographers surmount their own ethnocentrism through multicultural experiences that allow them to reach a higher level of generality, away from culture-bound attitudes and specificities towards broader dispositions. Even so, to maintain some degree of objectivity, it was thought important to avoid any evaluative intrusions into one's ethnographic efforts. However, as Bennett notes,

> The relativist view may be methodologically sound as a rule for the ethnologist to follow to avoid bias, but it makes little sense from the standpoint of problems of human existence, most of which are moral and which require judgments of good and bad, evil and benevolent (Bennett 1998, 361–2).

How Should We Study Well-Being through Culture?

So what standard or values do we use to define cultural well-being? Are we anthropologists to go out into the world to make pronouncements about what is good or bad about a society? After all, that is what missionaries do, and the results are mixed, to say the least. However, if we have benefited from the experience of living in societies alien to those in which we grew up, if we have had a wide range of ethnographic experience along with graduate training, we may have (to some extent at least) liberated ourselves from many of our own cultural demons and prejudices. But can we count on that kind of supracultural awareness? It is one thing to observe people starving, impoverished, or suffering from war trauma, and describe the obviously low level of well-being among them. It is another thing, however, to notice more subtle effects among people who are in less dire straits, or simply to make intuitive judgments on values among broad categories of groups, be they Muslim, Japanese, American, or any other. Do we need to have a theory of well-being or do we just add the topic of well-being to our ethnographic agenda and start writing? Answering that question takes us back to another question: what do we want anthropology to be—one of the sciences, one of the humanities, or some combination of the two? If we think anthropology ought to be a science, we should be concerned with matters of objectivity and ethnographic validity. These are matters that have been the subject of much debate in the past: the Lewis-Redfield differences over the description of Tepotzlan; the Mead-Freeman controversy over accuracy in Samoan ethnography; the dispute over Colin Turnbull's characterization of the Ik; and the emic-etic distinction that similar disagreements led to the 1960s and 1970s. If, on the other hand, we think that anthropology should be one of the humanities, the focus shifts to matters of responsibility toward one's ethnographic subjects, or to the wider context covered by social theorists from Marx, Durkheim, and Weber to Habermas and Foucault; one leans toward sociological, economic, and political issues, including the role and influence of investigators themselves, and to philosophical issues relating to these matters. Fortunately we don't legislate these matters in anthropology. It all depends on the ethnographer, the situation, and what the broader social needs might be.

Let's take the broader social needs for a moment. When anthropologists see the egregious mistakes in foreign policies that arise from a stultifying ignorance of the anthropology of regions, ethnicities, and religions around the world, we ask, "Why don't governments consult anthropologists?" Are anthropologists less equipped theoretically or ethnographically than other social scientists to take on advisory roles? Look at economics. There is an enormous input of advice to governments; but usually the input solicited, or hired, represents branches of the discipline, or individuals, that are most friendly to the ideology of whatever administration is in power. In short, there is a lot of politics in economics. Can we say that there are fewer political interests in anthropology? That question brings us back to the matter of objectivity. There are two paths anthropologists take toward greater objectivity: (1) our concern for the native point of view in an ethnography-based approach, and (2) a theory that has some claim to universal validity as, for example, one rooted in established biological principles.

As for (1), the fallback position for ethnographers is to ask the natives themselves what they think, or believe. That would mean some assessment of how representative each answer might be for whatever group is being described, which brings us eventually to a statistical approach. It also can bring us to a network approach, where we can study the relationships and features characteristic of that network. But why can't statistics and network analyses be interlarded with a more humanized, contextual approach as well? We can use the numbers and interpersonal network relations as a guide for open-ended questions to ask some of the subjects themselves. Oral narrative distributional analyses (Colby 1973; 1975), statistical approaches (Colby et al. 2003), and network analysis (White and Johansen 2005) need not be mutually exclusive with traditional, contextualized ethnography.

Short of these more formal or systematic approaches, the ethnographer must rely on his or her own perspicacity and implicit ideas about what increases or decreases cultural well-being. This returns us to the same questions that have haunted ethnography from its beginning. How might we as ethnographers assess the needs of our subjects and how might we, as outsiders but often with knowledge, technology, and facilities not available to those we study, help out as well as simply describe?

As ethnographers, most of us have provided some form of assistance to friends among the people we study. Often it includes transportation, such as driving a sick child to a medical facility, or it might include assisting in some educational form or in any number of other ways. What happens, however, when we, as ethnographers, see the wider problems that impact the society we study? These are difficult matters and sometimes there may not be all that much difference between anthropologists and activists who address injustices that clearly are perpetrated at higher national and international levels.

When writings get closer to actuality, to naming names and citing events, as in the works of Noam Chomsky, Howard Zinn, Arundhati Roy, Amy Goodman, and numerous other social critics, there is less theory to chew on and simply a compilation of facts concerning specific policies, events, and institutions. These writings are close to being ethnographies themselves, albeit ethnographic descriptions of policy consequences in a highly explicit sense of what is just and democratic versus what is hypocritical, dishonest, or self-serving. In any case, these writings have an explicit concern with well-being. Such writings relate in different ways to academic disciplines. Zinn sees his roles as historian and activist as one and the same. Chomsky, on the other hand, sees no connection between his activist writings and his role as linguist. What, in fact, are the differences between an ethnographic report on the well-being of some local situation and the writings of activists in some other category? Do we anthropologists really have something unique to share with the world? Do we have greater credibility because of our presumed cultural sensitivities? One of the problems with politics is that an observation pointing unambiguously to a wrongdoing is treated as a biased political opinion by the wrongdoer. We are living in an age where the pros and cons of torture are discussed by two talking heads on television as if each side were balanced in terms of morality. Perhaps ethnographers have more credibility than reporters and activist critics because they don't roil the waters. If they do, however—if they point to poverty and its causes in a region, for example—will they be treated as lacking in science because of political bias?

If one chooses to reveal what otherwise would remain hidden, how far up the chain of command of corporate or government behavior does one go? Will the processes of globalization (as influenced by the World Bank, the IMF, and other powerful entities) require that ethnographers, in order to write a full description of what is impacting well-being in their local area, bring national and international institutions under their purview as well, and from those institutions the social forces that created and maintain them? Any serious ethnography of the entire process would have to range from top-level economic forces down to the impact of their policies on the grass roots under the close eye of the ethnographer. Those top-level forces have a large component of sheer greed and drive for dominance cloaked in a legitimizing rhetoric and ideology. If that is the case, at the higher levels of investigation one would have to become an investigative reporter, seeking out textual materials in the form of memos, press statements, and books, including books by whistle blowers for the whole enterprise (Perkins 2004). Such activity is usually is considered off-limits to the anthropological enterprise. If we look at past studies of cultural well-being, we rarely see any disturbing of the political waters. But in the view of some observers, a disturbing of the waters is becoming increasingly necessary because hierarchical wealth-based connections are so often globally harmful in their consequences, and possibly irreversible.

A Brief History of Past Studies of Cultural Well-Being

Issues of cultural well-being and cultural pathology have been addressed in the past, but such attempts have not been widespread and are limited to only a few anthropologists, each with a different approach. Nevertheless, they are noteworthy and illustrate different approaches within the discipline.

Ruth Benedict's concern for prosocial values and behavior led to a concept she called "cultural synergy." At its simplest characterization, Benedict's ideas of cultural synergy emphasized cooperative and socially facilitative behavior—in currently popular terms, she meant a culture where most behavior was win-win, rather than win-lose. Sadly, her work was not taken up in anthropology and she dropped the idea herself to do other work. However, one of her students, Abraham Maslow, gained attention in psychology with his extension of her cultural synergy idea into the field of personality study. By applying Benedict's cultural synergy to individuals, in addition to his own original work, Maslow came to the idea of the "self-actualized" personality (1950).

Benedict's ideas about cultural synergy made intuitive good sense, but they lacked a full-length ethnographic treatment illustrating how her theory translated into actual ethnographic observation. She instead used scattered examples. Furthermore, some of her illustrations from ethnographies of societies she did not have first-hand acquaintance with were themselves ethnographically weak. In fairness to Benedict, however, all we are going on are lecture notes. She did not follow up on it, and Maslow, even though doing fieldwork among the Blackfeet in Canada, did not see how to deal with cultural synergy in any broad way. It was much easier, he found, to look at individuals and their personalities and values.

Raoul Naroll (1983) offered a more theoretically developed and testable approach, based on a cross-cultural viewpoint. Furthermore, he was the first anthropologist to address the problem of cultural well-being and pathology by means of what historians of science call a "theoretical program" (Kuhn 1970; Lakatos 1970) involving tests of hypotheses. The program focuses on what Naroll called "core values" and the review of social indicators along with a review of the state of the social sciences generally. Finally, after the crucial step of testing theory, Naroll went beyond this, to proposing actions to cope with problems identified in those tests.

Naroll's approach was to choose ten personal and family troubles studied cross-culturally: alcoholism, suicide, family disorganization, child abuse, juvenile delinquency, neglect of the elderly, sex roles, sexual frustration, and mental illness. These troubles could be studied through a constellation of social indicators, "scoreboards" he called them, which can give a general idea of how entire nations are coming along. Even with social indicator scoreboards, however, there is no way to deal with the dynamics that result in those indicators alone. A theory of well-being based on the kind of social indicators Naroll and sociologists usually use would have to include biological connections to well-being, child-rearing practices, institutional policies relating to economics, education, and a host of other areas. Actual ethnographic study in the field would be the ultimate, truly grassroots approach for arriving at a better contextual understanding of the dynamics that result in indicator scores. Finally, Naroll's moral categories (e.g., peace, order, and tolerance of diversity) were selected intuitively—hence, from a theoretical perspective, arbitrarily. There also is an assumption in Naroll's writings of cultural evolutionary progress (with pain and problems along the way). That assumption may be understandable for the times in which he wrote, but today seems less certain given the present world situation with all its vulnerabilities and misfortunes extending to many millions.

We have examined theory-based approaches to well-being and pathology; let us now turn to ethnography-based approaches. Oscar Lewis (1959, 1961, 1966) described a culture of poverty in the slums of cities around the world that, once started, became a self-perpetuating patho-

logical culture. Its characteristics were authoritarian attitudes and behavior, violence, lack of family solidarity, focus on instant gratification,
male abandonment, crowded living quarters, early awareness of sex,
and a fatalistic or cynical world view. Lewis raised hackles among some
of the politically correct element in anthropology. The whole idea of
a self-perpetuating loop or of a pathology of culture did not sit well
with a culturally relativistic stance. Since Lewis' work was primarily
descriptive, there was no explicit theoretical basis that could generate
testable hypotheses. Nevertheless, his ethnographies have had wide
readership and did much to alert the general public to the social and
cultural problems of extreme poverty.

Very interesting and useful, but less systematic and not theoretical,
is Robert Edgerton's *Sick Societies* (1992). This is a tour de force, a com-
pendium of every conceivable type of maladaptation an anthropologist
might encounter. The results of those maladaptations run the gamut
from alienation, despair, deprivation, fear, and hunger to sickness and
death. He argues that all societies have some beliefs and practices that
may be maladaptive, whether for everyone in the society or for some
of its members. Yet he holds to a conventional concept of culture, one
that draws a line around people who are inside the culture (and hence
might try to initiate changes) as opposed to outsiders, who should not
do anything to help except, perhaps, to serve as teachers or advisors to
members of "the culture":

> A scholarly discipline that can illuminate the sources of these kinds of
> human misery should command a large following, and with better under-
> standing of the sources of maladaptation may come means of reducing
> human suffering. We have no mandate to change other cultures because
> we find that some of their beliefs or practices are harmful to them, but
> we do have an obligation to understand and, when possible, to teach
> (Edgerton 1992, 208).

A very different approach is to be found in Jules Henry's book, *Culture Against Man* (1969), where he characterized aspects of American
culture as pathological. This interesting ethnographic approach to American society did not receive a lot of attention after the initial reviews because, I suspect, anthropologists didn't know just where or how to place
Henry's approach in the prevailing scheme of things anthropological.

There are undoubtedly other instances of anthropological concern
with well-being in the course of ethnographic research. Martin Orans
(1981), for example, has taken a dynamic approach to self-reported happiness as it relates to economic institutions and social ranking. Indeed,
any time major culture changes occur in an area under ethnographic attention, the evaluative element very often comes in: Who benefits from

the change? What brought about the change? George Appell suggests that with the kinds of massive changes that some populations undergo today, there develops a sense of bereavement from a past that no longer exists. He describes this as a "social separation syndrome" (1980).

After reviewing these past attempts at treating well-being, I suspect that the present book represents a major change, a tipping point of sorts within anthropology. When we compare the number of anthropologists in a single volume here to the sparseness of anthropologists in the previous century who were concerned with some form of cultural well-being, it is most encouraging. Those earlier studies were all by lone individuals. They did not represent a school, or tradition, or even any particularly influential theoretical program. Benedict's ideas did live in a way through Maslow's self-actualization writings, and Oscar Lewis had a wide reading public but has seldom been cited by anthropologists in recent generations. The others mentioned were similarly not followed by any significant number of ethnographers. To be sure, the present book does not represent a school or movement, but the fact that so many authors see their contributions as falling under the well-being tent suggests that what is different between now and the earlier history of well-being studies is that the zeitgeist is calling for it, and some of us are responding. The diversity of approaches in these chapters is in itself a strength and a sign of a broad change of orientation in the discipline.

The audience for studies of cultural well-being and pathology goes well beyond the anthropological profession. The great proliferation of NGOs and relief agencies show that there are hundreds of thousands of people willing to devote their lives to improving some small part of the world even at a low income level, or at home willing to go into an underpaid teaching profession to help children grow intellectually and morally. In short, I see the field of ethnographic attention to well-being as covering an enormous range of human endeavors extending well beyond card-carrying anthropologists. The world is desperately in need of more ethnographies of every type, especially those that give a full contextual description, that tell it like it is, whether they are written by anthropologists or by other investigators seeking, in a sophisticated and culturally sensitive way, to make the world a better place.

Let me explain this with my own example and history. My choice of an abiding theoretical program focusing on well-being began shortly after my ethnographic studies of the Ixil Maya of Guatemala. In the early 1980s, Guatemalan troops with US-trained officers were battling insurgents, Indian and Hispanic, in the lowlands of Guatemala and in the Ixil "triangle." The troops massacred entire hamlets and villages, men, women and children. Death squads were torturing and executing. Word about these atrocities among the Ixil and other Maya groups was not getting out to the rest of the world. I published letters in the *Los Angeles Times* and the *Wall Street Journal* and started a book about what was happening, essentially an ethnography of a war, but the more I learned the more it became evident that the ultimate cause was the political culture of foreign nations, most especially my own. So I had to make a choice: either devote the entire future to working on a theory of cultural pathology and well-being, or document what was happening among the people I already had been studying. Others came to the area and began studies in the Ixil triangle (Stoll 1993) and elsewhere in Guatemala. The word was getting out. With that responsibility covered, I chose the theoretical rather than the ethnographic approach. Elsewhere I have published a condensation of work during the ensuing twenty-five years in the study of cultural well-being and cultural pathology. It has included the theoretical generation of statements and the testing of those statements on students, and different ethnic and age groups in Orange County, California, some of it supported by a grant from the National Institute on Aging (Colby 1987, 2003; Colby et al. 2003). It also has included my research among the Ixil. I will start with the chief theoretical problem I thought had to be solved as the basis for such a theoretical program—the units of cultural analysis.

Theorizing Culture as "Self-world"

Freud's impasse was due to the prevailing ideas about culture, ideas that continue to dominate the meaning of culture even today. If one is to get around Freud's impasse, there has to be a revision in the conventional way culture is viewed. The first step is to deal with the three chief problems with conventional culture theory as it is currently used in anthropology. The first of these three problems is already partially attended to by the view of culture held among cognitive anthropologists (most explicitly by Ward Goodenough [1996]) and some psychological anthropologists (Schwartz 1978). This is the locus of culture—where does culture reside (if anywhere)? Cognitive anthropologists and many psychological anthropologists now see that locus as in people's heads. But actually that is only a partial solution, as I will get to below.

The second problem is the lack of a biological connection, when obviously there is a powerful connection between culture and our biology. The third problem is the assumption of cultural relativism. I will briefly expand on the first below and then develop solutions to the other two problems.

The problem of location can be addressed through the concept of "self-world." With the increasing complexity of society today, with migrations, refugees, and entire businesses moving across national boundaries, the superorganic view of culture—whether in the small (where the world is populated with a great number of "cultures" as count nouns) or in the large (where *culture* is used as a mass noun equivalent to *civilization*)—is inadequate, as earlier discussed. One way to deal with the location problem is to distinguish between schemas inside our heads, and culture patterns observed in our surroundings. In such a tandem view, we focus on the interchange between schemas and patterns in terms of a self-world unit of analysis. Culture patterns are located in behavior and in the built environment. The vehicles for these patterns are people and material culture. With schemas to perceive patterns as they come through to the mind, a major division is within the brain—a division between (1) the perceptual mechanisms that allow us to recognize patterns observed in the outside world and replicate them or modify them in our own thinking and (2) the effecting of behavior through effector schemas in the mind. The second, quite obvious division is simply between mind and the cultural patterns perceived to exist in the surrounding world.

By focusing on culture as a process between mind and surrounding world, culture is thus a process, an interacting tandem of schemas in the mind and patterns in the outside world. In sum, cultural patterns are carried by vehicles: other humans, as expressed in what they say and do; artifacts (including spoken words and symbol-laden artifacts like books); and the built environment.

As long as "the culture" is the unit of analysis, we can never get to cultural dynamics. If we seek to describe "a culture" as a unit, a set of values in some coherent configuration, we will miss the effects of conflicts and disharmonies within the society that holds that "culture." Furthermore, we will miss the crosscurrents from cultural patterns that originate outside the "culture." This is particularly the case with the globalization of culture through the media and through economic effects.

In this emerging global age, my Ixil Maya assistant, Shas, can walk down the road from his house to the center of his village in the western mountains of Guatemala and for a small fee, log onto the internet and send me e-mail, whereas during my first visit to the area many years ago, there was not even a television set anywhere in the village. On my third trip in the 1970s, there was one television set in the town hall, which when I watched, was presenting the Dick van Dyke show (popular in the US in the 1960s) dubbed in Spanish. So obviously we cannot continue with the old conventional view of culture as a bounded entity, coinciding with tribe, island, or even language, whether occupying a narrowly delimited space or characterizing an entire nation, religion, or civilization. Nor can we accept the superorganic assumptions that culture and biology are totally separate. That does not mean giving up on culture as a viable concept. Clearly we cannot do without culture; we just need a different view of culture and different units of cultural analysis.

Maslow went from Ruth Benedict's cultural synergy to individual psychology because there was just no way to deal with an entire "culture" as conceptualized during Benedict's time. However we can shift culture theory toward the person with yet another unit, the self-world, similar in some respects to von Uexkull's *Umwelt* (1957). Von Uexkull describes his unit in terms of perceptors and effectors in studies of animal behavior: "All that a subject perceives becomes his perceptual world and all that he does, his effector world. Perceptual and effector worlds together form a closed unit" (1957, 6). We can do the same. With the self-world as the basic unit of cultural analysis, we are better able to examine the dynamics at work within a society of any type, of any ethnic, ideological, religious, or language mix. At the same time, to be more rigorous, individuals can be linked to other individuals as nodes in social networks with different bases of linkages (friendship, contact frequency, profession, birth origin, language, professed values, and so on). Social networks, in turn, can be referred to in casual ethnographic text, on some observational basis, or more precisely through computers, as in formal network analysis.

Within the self-world, the chief division is essentially that between the perception of patterns and the matching of those patterns with schemas (or schemata). The self-world thus consists of the self and two surrounds: the immediate surround of first-hand experience, and a second surround of hearsay or indirect experience (i.e., through accounts of someone else's experience) and in the print and electronic world, primarily the public figures encountered through television and newsprint. The self-world is a convenient construct for trying to represent inner views, if need be, through the usual procedures of interviewing and observation as well as through questionnaires, sentence completion test, TATs, autobiographies, and diary records, not to mention recordings of actual events through video and photos. With the individual person at the center of the self-world, the individual's cognitive schemas, motivations, emotions, values, and attitudes as well as the physical body are all part of the mix.

The beginnings of a theory of well-being and adaptive potential distinguish within the self-world three realms of concern. Today neuropsychological evidence suggests neural bases for this tripartite division (Colby 2003), but much earlier Malinowski used it in organizing how he thought about culture and its institutions. I characterize this tripartite division as follows: First is the natural and cultural ecology as perceived and as accessed by the self. It also covers one's own biology and physical body. Included further in this realm is the ecological inheritance biologists speak about when discussing niche construction of animals (leaf cutter ants and their earth constructions, beavers and their dams) and of course for humans that also means the built environment. I describe this as the *material or biophysical realm*. Second is the *interpersonal realm* where the individual normally operates in face-to-face interactions with other people. I have used the term *interpersonal* rather than *social* to emphasize that this realm is primarily an interactive one between persons, and only secondarily does it go to a wider coverage of everything else that is social, which often includes a more abstract representation than simply interpersonal interactions. Third and last, there is the *symbolic realm* involving higher-order thinking and language and all forms of symbolic behavior.

A similar tripartite division of realms was made by Malinowski (1960, 136) when he said that culture originated from an integration of three lines of development:

> 1). "the ability to recognize instrumental objects, the appreciation of their technical efficiency, and their value, that is, their place in the purposive sequence" (i.e., enhancing one's ability to wrest a living in the nonsocial material and biological realm)
>
> 2). "the formation of social bonds" (the interpersonal realm)
>
> 3). "the appearance of symbolism" (the symbolic realm)

In each of these three realms I have developed measures of what I describe as conditions of adaptive potential. Measures in the material and interpersonal realms have inversely correlated with measures of physical and mental symptoms. This shows a direct linkage to biology, and through that to evolutionary theory (Colby 2003). At the moment, my measures for conditions in the symbolic realm are undergoing major revisions, going beyond the originally postulated conditions of creativity and metaknowledge to include goal orchestration and the separate components and processes involved with invention and creative behavior. So, until more exploratory research is completed for conditions in the symbolic realm, tests of the theory will be based on conditions in the material and interpersonal realms. The results of those tests are reported elsewhere (Colby 1987, 2003; Colby et al. 2003). Here, I will briefly describe the history and current exploratory findings with the symbolic realm.

I began by postulating creativity as the primary condition of adaptive potential in this realm. The link to evolution is obvious, for it is through creative endeavors that humans and human culture have advanced to where we are today. However, creativity is exceedingly hard to measure, particularly with the kind of questionnaire that I have successfully used with the first two realms. It turned out that in regression analyses, my measures of creativity did not add to the power of my regression analyses in the company of my measures in the first two realms. Exploratory analyses suggested that this is because the symbolic realm sits atop the material and interpersonal realms and in many ways is a more abstract mirroring of those first two realms. I have begun to think more in terms of findings concerning neurological development, particularly the evolutionarily more recent prefrontal cortices. A key element to be measured in this area is likely to be the ability to delay instant gratification. That means decisions and behavior in keeping with cultural appropriateness. Forethought often suggests that for some behaviors there are situational preconditions where often a later time for some behavioral action would be more beneficial for the long-term success of the individual.

In addition to timing is consistency of values and sense of self. Consistency includes the ability to see connections and to bring cultural elements and patterns into coherent relationships for a more meaningful and successful life. I now see the primary condition of adaptive potential in the symbolic realm to be coherence and timing, with subcategories of coherence-building processes (such as creative processing and goal orchestration). I have not yet been able to fully develop a way to measure this broad and very subtle mix of cognition and valence (the marking of goals with past and imagined future emotional experiences), and so I leave that aside here while awaiting a test of measures for conditions in the symbolic realm along the lines I have just sketched out.

It is the testing of adaptive potential theory that returns us to the crucial aspect of biology and evolution. The conventional view of culture, especially the ignoring of the fundamental linkage that exists between biology and culture, precludes a proper attention to emotions, the basis out of which value systems emerge. Too long have developmental and evolutionary biology been regarded as irrelevant to cultural processes. Yet a moment's reflection confirms that culture is intimately linked to biology in both these fields, not the least of which is through emotional systems of neuronal wiring and hormonal infusions, which surely affect our values as well as our cultural experiences.

Is a Measure of Well-Being Possible or Desirable?

So, finally, we return to the question in the title. At the simplest level, we can always ask the people we interview how happy they are, what makes them happy, and what makes them unhappy. Simple and obvious though it may be, such questions can be enormously productive. Diener studies responses to questions on happiness as "subjective well-being" (Diener and Suh 2000). Many other techniques are possible. William Dressler inventoried the material culture in people's houses and rated individuals in those houses according to the kind of lifestyle aspirations represented by those material artifacts. Adding other variables, such as income, he came up with a measure of lifestyle incongruity. The more the incongruity, the higher the blood pressure, and for young people, the more likely was there to be depression (Dressler 1990, 1991). Since biology and culture are intimately related, these connections can be the source of interesting clues to biocultural dynamics that are moving beneath the surface of explicit recognition. When these currents involve stress, they take a toll on the body and therefore lower the probability of an extended life span.

With the adaptive potential measure (Colby 2003), preliminary tests in the material and interpersonal realms support the statement that the greater the score on adaptive potential, the fewer the symptoms of physical and mental ill health. These and similar measures can be used to test the theory that human values that promote quiescent (parasympathetic) bodily states promote longevity and survival and hence link core cultural values to our biology and to evolutionary theory as well as to other aspects of culture in a coherent and meaningful way.

There can be many different ways to measure adaptive potential. I used questionnaires together with thematic apperception stimuli (pictures) to get spontaneous texts from the individuals in the sample (Colby et al. 2003). It is my hope that a system of content analysis might also be applied in tests of the theory. If the theory seems to be intuitively a sensible theory, one can simply use the theory as a new kind of *Notes and Queries* during ethnographic study, as a guide to questions and directions one might want to use in interviews, the preferred technique of most ethnographers, in addition to direct observations and participant observation.

Earlier I argued that a major support for cultural relativism was that it obviated value judgments on the part of the ethnographer, and hence an ethnography that eschewed any value judgments or political commentary on the situation of the people being described was more likely to be treated as objective, or scientific. This rationale no longer holds.

There are many obvious uses of a truly objective theory of well-being. Testing for adaptive potential or for some general measure of well-being, for example, can provide a form of feedback after some ameliorative intervention for a society, or after some historical change. Moving away from subjective, opinion-based ideas can lessen the intrusion of politically motivated arguments, to something that is more objective and hence less influenced by vested interests and idiosyncrasies.

One of the arguments brought forward in postmodern anthropology was that the ethnographer cannot be completely immune to making value judgments, and indeed should be willing to actively assist in the well-being of those being studied, often an assistance going beyond local help to activism at some higher level. Perhaps the best analogy is with health. Doctors try to improve the health of their patients and they can be objective in describing what is good health and what is bad health. At higher levels, however, activism among physicians takes a different form: Doctors Without Borders, Physicians for Social Responsibility, etc. Since those higher levels go beyond proximal causes of ill health, they bring medical people directly up against government and corporate policies that may be impacting the health of people. The major area of difficulty, of course, is the equation of high adaptive potential with liberal or progressive politics and low adaptive potential with authoritarianism and right-wing fundamentalist groups in any religion. The theory was developed out of a thought experiment, tested, and supported. It was only later that I recognized how close the conditions of high adaptive potential were correlated with real democracy, and how low adaptive potential links to repression and sham democracy. Can anyone seriously argue against high affiliation, prosocial autonomy, trust, and altruism—all conditions of high adaptive potential in the interpersonal realm? When the consequences of public or foreign policy are breaking down those conditions at home and abroad, it is time to think about a cultural well-being audit just as economists look to and audit the economic well-being of a society.

References

Appell, George N. 1980. "The Social Separation Syndrome." *Survival International Review* 5, no. 1 (29): 13–15.

Bennett, John W. 1998. *Classic Anthropology: Critical Essays, 1944–1996.* New Brunswick, NJ: Transaction Publishers.

Colby, Benjamin N. 1973. "A Partial Grammar of Eskimo Folktales." *American Anthropologist* 75 (3): 645–62.

———. 1975. "Culture Grammars." *Science* 187 (4180): 913–19.

————. 1987. "Well-being: A Theoretical Program." *American Anthropologist* 89 (4): 879–95.

————. 2003. "Toward a Theory of Culture and Adaptive Potential." *Human Complex Systems. Mathematical Anthropology and Culture Theory: An International Journal* 1 (3): 1–53.

Colby, Benjamin. N., Kathryn Azevedo, and Carmella C. Moore. 2003. "The Influence of Adaptive Potential on Proximate Mechanisms of Natural Selection." *Mathematical Anthropology and Culture Theory: An International Journal* 1 (3): 1–24.

Diener, Ed and Eunkook M. Suh. 2000. *Culture and Subjective Well-Being.* Cambridge, MA: MIT Press.

Dressler, William W. 1990. "Lifestyle, Stress, and Blood Pressure in a Southern Black Community." *Psychosomatic Medicine* 52: 182–98.

————. 1991. *Stress and Adaptation in the Context of Culture: Depression in a Southern Black Community.* Albany, NY: State University of New York Press.

Edgerton, Robert B. 1992. *Sick Societies: Challenging the Myth of Primitive Harmony.* New York: The Free Press.

Freud, Sigmund 1961 [1930]. *Civilization and Its Discontents.* Trans. James Strachey. New York and London: W.W. Norton.

Goodenough, Ward. 1996. "Culture." In *Encyclopedia of Cultural Anthropology,* ed. David Levinson and Melvin Ember, 291–99. New York: Henry Holt & Co.

Henry, Jules. 1969. *Culture Against Man.* New York: Random House.

Kuhn, Thomas S. 1970. *The Structure of Scientific Revolutions,* 2 vols. 2nd, enlarged ed., *International Encyclopedia of Unified Science,* ed. Otto Neurath vol. 2. Chicago: University of Chicago Press.

Lakatos, Imre. 1970. "Falsification and the Methodology of Scientific Research Programmes." In *Criticism and the Growth of Knowledge,* ed. I. Lakatos and A Musgrave. Cambridge: Cambridge University Press.

Lewis, Oscar. 1959. *Five Families: Mexican Case Studies in the Culture of Poverty.* New York: Basic Books.

————. 1961. *The Children of Sanchez.* New York: Random House.

————. 1966. *La Vida: A Puerto Rican Family in the Culture of Poverty—San Juan and New York.* New York: Random House.

Malinowski, Bronislaw. 1960. *A Scientific Theory of Culture and Other Essays.* New York: Oxford University Press.

Maslow, Abraham H. 1950. *Self-Actualizing People: A Study of Psychological Health.* New York: Grune and Stratton.

Naroll, Raoul. 1983. *The Moral Order: An Introduction to the Human Situation.* Beverly Hills, CA: Sage Publications.

Orans, Martin. 1981. "Hierarchy and Happiness in a Western Samoan Community." In *Social Inequality; Comparative and Developmental Approaches,* ed. G.D. Berreman. New York: Academic Press.

Perkins, John. 2004. *Confessions of an Economic Hit Man.* San Francisco: Berrett-Koehler Publishers.

Schwartz, Theodore. 1978. "Where Is the Culture? Personality as the Distributive Locus of Culture." In *The Making of Psychological Anthropology,* ed. G.D. Spindler. Berkeley: University of California Press.

Stoll, David. 1993. *Between Two Armies in the Ixil Towns of Guatemala*. New York: Columbia University Press.

von Uexkull, Jakob. 1957. "A Stroll through the Worlds of Animals and Men: A Picture Book of Invisible Worlds." In *Instinctive Behavior: The Development of a Modern Concept*, ed. Claire H. Schiller. New York: International Universities Press.

White, Douglas R. and Ulla Johansen. 2005. *Network Analysis and Ethnographic Problems: Process Models of a Turkish Nomad Clan*. Oxford, Boston, Lexington Press.

PART TWO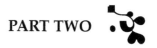

WELL-BEING IN SMALL-SCALE SOCIETIES

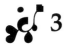 3

WELL-BEING AMONG THE MATSIGENKA OF THE PERUVIAN AMAZON
Health, Missions, Oil, and "Progress"
Carolina Izquierdo

> We used to think it was good to have a nice, clean house. We worked in the gardens, we made things . … We just lived. … You lived with your wife, without fighting, in peace. People came and visited. Now it's not enough. If a man wants a woman he just tells her, "Look, I have a watch" or "Look at my radio. I have all these things." But this is deceit. When they live together, the man doesn't even give her good food. Before, we didn't deceive. We just said, "Look, I'm a good hunter." (Alberto, a Matsigenka man)

In this chapter I discuss the relationship between biomedical, individual, and societal assessments of well-being among the Matsigenka of the Peruvian Amazon, as they seek to preserve their senses of wellness despite their rapidly changing social and economic environment. Matsigenka senses of well-being give us insight into a horticultural/hunter-gatherer society that has only recently been in frequent contact with the larger world. The Matsigenka are now experiencing the full impact of globalization in their daily lives, for under their territory lies one of the largest natural gas reserves in Latin America, currently being extracted by multinational companies. My research indicates that despite objective measures that show people getting "healthier," the Matsigenka feel that their well-being is in drastic decline.[1] This shows that well-being is something much more than the conditions that doctors and medical personnel can measure through physiological examinations. Well-being is a matter of how individuals feel about themselves in their society, in a situation of uncertain future survival.

The concept of well-being[2] presents serious difficulties for researchers in all disciplines in that it can be very broadly defined, resulting in the use of unclear methodologies and definitions, and making it very difficult to compare cross-culturally. One of the fundamental dilemmas we face when trying to define and study well-being among different groups is that even if we can agree that it is human nature to strive for well-being in terms of general fulfillment, there is still a problem in determining which ideals people are using to evaluate their well-being. Well-being may be envisioned as an individual venture or conceived of as existing in realms beyond the self, and may involve projection of the values of the past, or of the values of an emergent future. Studies have, for the most part, equated well-being with individuals' judgments about life satisfaction as a "global assessment of a person's quality of life according to his own chosen criteria" (Diener 1996, 543). But as Christopher points out, "this approach is directly linked to certain Western individualistic assumptions and values—or moral visions" (1999, 143). The very notion of "assessing" a person's well-being assumes that well-being is not taken for granted (see Adelson 2000), that its fluctuations can be measured in some way, and that these measurements have meaning. This individualistic concept of assessment also implies that a person is both capable of and adept at observing his or her feelings, and able to separate his or her state of mind from the surrounding environment. Furthermore, if well-being can be measured and assessed, it can also be improved. Some sense of the production of well-being is implied in societies that stress individual agency optimizing personal life satisfaction, however that may be measured. At the same time, some degree of unproductiveness is associated with those who do not achieve a sense of well-being.

Among the Matsigenka, well-being is seen as being in decline: the Matsigenka behold a breakdown of the body and the society, an existential crisis wherein the individual and close kin search for a culturally coherent explanation for their distress (violation of cultural taboos, for example, or having been stingy with someone). The Matsigenka have no word that directly translates into English as *health, well-being,* or *wellness* or to the equivalent in Spanish such as *salud,* which directly translates into "health." For example, among the Matsigenka, personal health is translated as "taking care of one's body" (*aneginteigakerora ashiegi avatsaegi*), indicating the importance the Matsigenka give to cleanliness and purity of the body. Perhaps closest to *well-being* is the concept of *shinetagantsi,* most commonly translated as "happiness" or "becoming happy," which embodies ideas and ideals of what the Matsigenka consider the basic premise of a good life.

In this chapter I explore well-being for the Matsigenka through their own personal accounts, through insights that physical examinations provide, and through my observations while living with them. Within a historical context, I discuss socioculturally mediated experience and subjective expressions of what "the good life" feels like for the Matsigenka.

The Matsigenka in a Historical Context

This study draws on ethnographic research I conducted between 1996 and 2004. Although I visited most Matsigenka communities in the Lower Urubamba region, this research was carried out mainly in the Kamisea[3] community located along the Urubamba River. I also draw on previous research carried out by other scholars among the Matsigenka in the late 1960s, early 1970s, and 1980s in order to establish a longitudinal time-line to draw comparisons. The primary methods I used for data collection were participant observation, semistructured and open-ended interviews with most members of the community (the small-scale setting provided me the luxury of interviewing most people), and video recordings of everyday activities and interactions. Cognitive tasks, such as pile sorts and free listing, were used in order to elucidate theories of health and illness. I checked health post records, and physical medical examinations were conducted in collaboration with medical personnel working in the area (Izquierdo 2005).

The Matsigenka are an Arawakan-speaking people numbering be-tween ten and twelve thousand. They inhabit the regions of the Uru-bamba River and its tributaries, the Madre de Dios region, and Manu National Park in Peru.

The Matsigenka are a "family-level" society (A. Johnson 2003) who in the past lived in scattered nuclear family residences or hamlets, subsist-ing on a combination of fishing, foraging, and horticulture—primarily maize and manioc. Although subsistence and family organization re-main in place, in recent decades, communities have been established as permanent settlements under the direction of the Summer Institute of Linguistics (Protestant missionaries), organized around government-sponsored bilingual schools and health posts. Currently there are ap-proximately twenty Matsigenka communities in the Lower Urubamba region. Settlements initiated by missionaries have greatly changed the Matsigenka way of life. Up until recently, Matsigenka lacked the fea-tures of social organization common to villages, including formalized political structures, communal meeting places, and activities such as pan-tribal feasts. Land ownership and the control over resources such as excess food and goods were not sources of conflict, in stark contrast to the current situation. A history of sparse, mobile, and flexible social organization meant that the Matsigenka did not develop mechanisms other than flight to deal with individual or family conflict. Historically, the Matsigenka actively avoided contact with outsiders as a means of self-preservation. The 1950s were a frightening period for the Matsi-genka living in the Urubamba region. During the height of the slave

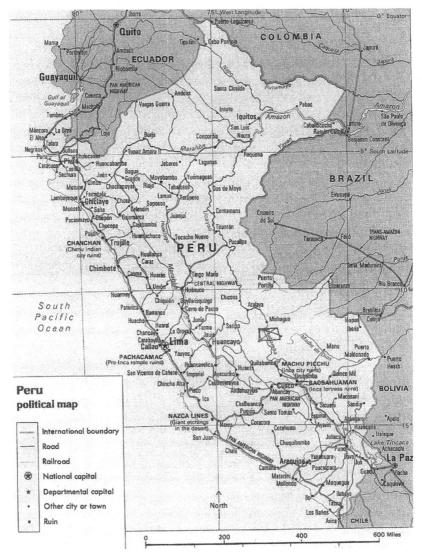

Figure 3.1 Map of Peru

trade, which lasted well into the 1950s, most fled with their families into the headwaters of the Kamisea River and others into the Picha and Parotori Rivers. But many Matsigenka were not so fortunate. Their tales of exploitation and subjugation during the period of the slave trade include accounts of murder.[4]

In the 1940s, as part of their world plan to disseminate the teachings of the Bible, missionaries employed by the Wycliff Bible Translators (SIL) came to Peru to translate the New Testament into all native languages. Evangelical missionaries embarked on this project with the messianic belief that once this monumental task had been completed, Christ would return to earth. While translating the Bible and learning local languages, missionaries sought to spread Christianity to the indigenous peoples with whom they came into contact. The Matsigenka, for the most part, were beyond the cultural reach of the missionaries, because they lived within the furthest depths of the Amazon. Their settlement pattern of scattered hamlets built away from the main rivers was well suited to guarantee some success in their escape. To reach them, missionaries had to labor to consolidate the dispersed local groups into larger settled communities. Although their main goal was to assimilate and evangelize the Matsigenka, their work also included the training of schoolteachers and health workers.

The Protestant evangelical church was instrumental in stamping out the cultural healing practices of Matsigenka shamans through wholesale demonization of their practices. Consequently, without shamans (*seripigari*) and with accusations of sorcery (*matsitagantsi*) on the rise in Kamisea, there are currently few alternatives for dealing with illnesses (*mantsigarintsi*) that do not respond to the limited biomedical treatment available, and may not even be recognized by health workers. The Matsigenka have found innovative remedies by incorporating a new category of "curers" (*itsimpokantavagetira*) into their ethnomedical system. Thus, a new class of "health professionals" has in a sense emerged, to address this need for culturally informed illness management: a social-spiritual expert, the curer. However, curers can only partially alleviate the sense of malaise and of ill-being felt by many Matsigenka today.

Currently, although outside education and health personnel live in Matsigenka communities, there is little effort to facilitate cultural understanding or exchange. Rather, visitors, government personnel, and agents of the media promulgate a nearly universal sentiment of disdain towards the *natives*—"nativos"—stressing instead the urgent need for cultural change. The *cambio* (change, "progress") that settlers and government representatives advocate is generally that of acculturation into mainstream Peruvian life. The pressure to change their culture and to make "progress" has provoked in the Matsigenka a justifiable fear about their future. The Matsigenka have grown increasingly agitated about the massive cultural changes derived from new settlement patterns and international development projects in their region, and face strong pressure to comply with the demands of economic development and the consequent social, spiritual, and cultural requirements of this development.

While indigenous peoples like the Matsigenka are asked to modern-
ize and change their traditional selves, they are at the same time expected to sell their indigenous exotic persona in order to participate in
eco-tourism aimed at attracting visitors for national profit (Izquierdo
and Casey 2003). Although the Matsigenka express general confusion
regarding their cultural identity and their religious identity in particular, due to missionary Christianization, they recognize some advantages to having been missionized. If not for missionaries, they would
still live scattered in the forest speaking only the Matsigenka language,
they sometimes say. Presently, in light of their recent dealings with
large oil corporations and government agencies, they feel that without
schools, they would be more vulnerable if they only spoke their language and lacked the organizational skills to help them deal with the
economic, social, and environmental decisions they face.

Today, multinational oil companies such as Plus Petrol are carrying
out a multimillion-dollar "Camisea Gas Project"[5] in the heart of Matsigenka territory. Despite the difficulties of oil and gas extraction, Plus
Petrol forged ahead with their project in the jungle. Barges and helicop-
ters hauling supplies up and down the Urubamba River have become a
common sight. In contrast to my first visit in 1996, when I encountered
few if any people other than the Matsigenka, the "Camisea Gas Project" has attracted not only laborers from other regions, but many international organizations providing input into health and environmental
services, and associated researchers and activists such as health specialists and environmentalists. Due to the magnitude of the gas extraction
operations in the area, many outsiders frequented Kamisea during my
fieldwork. The press arrived in the region as well, and, practically overnight, this remote region became headline news in distant Lima, Peru's
capital. The impact of these sudden changes has been directly felt in
terms of subsistence, demographics, and social organization, leading
the Matsigenka to view many aspects of foreign culture as having the
potential to cause illness, misfortune, and social disruption.

To my dismay, the international spotlight on the region has served
mainly to reinforce negative stereotypes about indigenous people. It was
all too common to hear comments that "these Indians" were lazy and
dirty. Similarly, outsiders attributed illness and misfortune among the
Matsigenka to ignorance and irresponsible reproduction, which were
felt to result in large families and "poverty." The general prescription
for their ills was to recommend that birth control be mandatory. Visitors and agents of the media promulgated a nearly universal sentiment
of disdain towards "natives." These outsiders were seemingly unaware
of their own ignorance in judging the purported backwardness of the

Matsigenka. I quote a health worker working among the Matsigenka: "I don't think they speak a real language. ... They just make noises and this is how they communicate. I will record them and see if there is any form of language in what they say." Ironically, my own experience among the Matsigenka showed me that they were much more "civilized" than many of the foreigners who came to "help" them. The *cambio* or change that settlers and government representatives advocated was generally that of acculturation, echoing similar notions expressed centuries earlier by missionaries. However, I found the attitudes of urban Mestizos and European Peruvians to be no harsher than similar ethnic and class-based hostility expressed elsewhere in Latin America; for example, in Chile where I am from and where I have worked extensively (Izquierdo 1995). I also highlight the fact that in addition to the hostility I witnessed and experienced from outside individuals and entities, I also met people—several anthropologists, health workers, company employees, and others—who cared deeply and wanted for the massive operation to benefit all involved. They stressed the importance of understanding the local environment and establishing good relationships with the Matsigenka people. The different interests among all the parties involved have been a difficult struggle for all.

Matsigenka Health/Well-Being and Their Contradictions

I earlier noted that Matsigenka perceptions of their well-being differ markedly from objective medical examinations results. I will now discuss this in more detail. In 1998 I collaborated with medical practitioners working in this area, where we tested a random sample of 104 individuals (out of a total population of 265 people). The health assessments here discussed incorporate physical examinations, analyses of blood samples for hemoglobin and serum proteins, and analyses of stool samples in order to assess parasite burden. These data were then compared to a similar study conducted twenty years previously with this community by Strongin (1982) as well as to an even earlier medical assessment conducted in 1968 (Weiseke 1968; Soto 1982). I do not use mortality or morbidity indices to describe the population, as there are no reliable statistical data. The health post in Kamisea dates back only to 1997, clearly not long enough to make claims about mortality rates over time.

Contrary to the Matsigenka's reports of decreased physical health, as I discuss below, physical examinations show that in 1998 the population in Kamisea seems to be in significantly better physical health than twenty to thirty years ago (Izquierdo 2005). For both males and females, proteins and hemoglobin were significantly higher in 1998 than in 1977. This seems due to better general nutrition, better hygiene, and perhaps to the introduction of Western healthcare and pharmaceuticals. Increased aerobic activity could also help explain lower pulses for men in Kamisea in recent years, which is congruent with men's reports of having to travel farther to hunt and cultivate gardens. Higher levels of hemoglobin indicate better nutritional status. We also see a significant decrease in parasites. One reason for this may be that Kamisea has improved its water supply, thanks to the installation of a large well four years ago, with faucets from which people now get their drinking water. This is much better than the previous practice of drinking water from the contaminated Urubamba River. In addition to improved sanitation facilities, including an expanded number of latrines and better management of waste, the community has benefited from public health education designed to prevent infectious and parasitic disease in new settlements such as Kamisea. It is still important to keep in mind that the initial formation of large settlements brought epidemics and disaster to native groups—resulting in a possible loss of up to two-thirds of native populations (Gade 1972)—which could have resulted in increased parasites and low protein levels. We have no way of knowing, as there are no physical examinations from that time period.

Baksh (1984) predicted that the main threat for the Matsigenka would be their physical health due to depletion of resources and diet. Although these threats are very real, I argue that social conflict engendered by settlement and outsiders is much more of a threat to the well-being of these communities than is competition for natural resources such as fish and game. As the next section will show, while physical health for the Matsigenka has shown improvement, they sense their well-being to have become dramatically worse.

The Matsigenka Life Cycle: Growing Up to Live Well

> To be happy, one must live in a place far away from Mestizos and away from flu and smallpox. Before, we didn't know how to wash dishes, we ate out of *pamocos* [coconut shells or calabashes used as bowls], we used monkey heads as spoons and we didn't have illnesses. We didn't have to boil water and we lived in peace. We were happy without having to wash our hands all the time. … Now health personnel come and say we have to wash our hands all the time, boil water for everything, and make latrines to be happy, but before we *were* happy. (Andrea, a twenty-five-year-old Matsigenka woman)

According to the Matsigenka I spoke with, well-being is linked to ideals about happiness, which are, in themselves, embedded in notions of productivity, goodness, and maintaining harmony with the social, physical, and spiritual environment. Socialization into these ideal or expected values and behaviors are strongly enforced since early childhood. The Matsigenka believe that a child's fate can be determined while in the mother's womb. Restrictive food practices and taboos are especially pronounced during pregnancy. Both parents observe special dietary rules as well as rules governing activity in order to ensure the well-being of the family as a whole; otherwise the results could include unwanted physical features as well as undesirable personality traits (e.g., stinginess, anger, laziness, dishonesty, and disrespect) in the developing fetus. Soon after a baby's birth, the parents return to their productive routines to exemplify collaboration and productivity. An individual is believed to exert his or her own will, as a fetus in the womb, during life and after death. These beliefs are manifest, for example, when parents of a dying child attribute the death to the baby's intent. I was told many times, as an infant was about to die, that the baby showed a lack of will to survive.

Children are cherished and protected by a network of family members and the community at large. Because kin are always nearby, children grow up with much attention and love. Both girls and boys are treated with the same love and care. The fact that the mother's sisters are referred to as classificatory mothers and father's brothers are classificatory fathers provides an expanded circle of relatives interested in the well-being of the child. This is manifested in the frequency with which they visit one another and in the extent of food sharing.

The need for competence, autonomy, and sociability are all basic tenets for a good life among the Matsigenka, and behavior that reinforces those feelings is believed to lead to lifelong feelings of well-being. Competence begins early in life, when children model and emulate the parents' activities in the home and in the gardens. Little girls do women's work while little boys do what their fathers and elders do. They acquire a high degree of competency by the time they reach their adolescent years. In the process, boys and girls slowly acquire autonomy through trial and error. Everybody has a clear idea of what one is supposed to be doing and how to behave. I was struck by how reluctant the Matsigenka were to judge or evaluate the actions of others, even children. I became very accustomed to hearing the phrases; "it's up to her," "it's up to him," "it's up to them," or "it's up to you." The Matsigenka are particularly careful with hearsay by including in the conversation whether the reported information was witnessed or told directly or whether it was gained by secondhand accounts. This caution serves to protect the speaker from being accused of gossip or deceit, behaviors that are destructive to community life and at the same time highly likely to be produced through accusations of sorcery.

Socialization of appropriate emotions and protection of the individual and the society are ensured by a variety of herbal treatments administered by parents and grandparents. There are clear cultural norms that govern emotions such as fear and anger. Fear is always mentioned by men and women as a source of vulnerability, an emotion to be strictly controlled lest one open oneself to illness or social marginalization. Likewise, anger is considered a dangerous emotion. Angry words or actions threaten the harmony of families and are especially threatening to the fragile balance of newly formed communities. Another core value of the Matsigenka is respect for communal and individual property, "not taking anything that doesn't belong to you" (they believe that Mestizo schoolteachers teach children to steal). Consequently they are suspicious of the value of education and are uncertain whom or what is responsible for their children's learning to steal, lack of respect, and becoming lazy.

Adult life is characterized by extreme self-sufficiency of the Matsigenka household and a balanced division of labor between husband and wife. The term for old age is *gatavaigetagantsi*, which translates literally as "to be done, to be satisfied after a long life," implying a sense of completion and fulfillment that contrasts with Western notions of old age as decay and decrepitude (Shepard 1999). The elderly are highly respected for their knowledge of medicinal plants, mythology, history, and folklore, and for their entertaining yarns about a past that was more difficult and yet easier in some ways, more treacherous, and more mysterious than life today (Izquierdo and Shepard 2003).

Although the Matsigenka idealize the forest as the place of their own origins, they also fear it for its mystical powers. This duality suggests that although the Matsigenka believe the boundaries between themselves, animals, nature, and the supernatural are easily crossed, they construct a cultural border against this invasive liminality by locating it in remote forests. There are dozens of songs about beautiful flowers and animals and even more folktales that describe in detail the lives and attributes of magical animals that live in the forest. Other folktales serve to codify and distinguish good behavior from bad. Allen Johnson describes the pervasive intentionality uniting all animate beings in the Matsigenka world and having souls capable of both harm and goodness (2003). The idea of every being having a purpose, self-will, and correct norms to follow is widely reflected in Matsigenka ideas of conflict avoidance, humble behavior, respect for privacy, and fears related to the will of others—their envy, greed, lust, or special powers. Right and wrong conduct is socialized early in childhood and there are tacit rules of behavior governing liminal periods in the life cycle, particularly illness, pregnancy, childbirth, and death.

The good spirits, or *Saankarite,* are said to live in remote high places in the rain forest, recognized as untouched by the incursions of modern life, and embody the ideals of a golden pastoral past. They are the creators of bliss and well-being. However, being in good graces with the *Saankarite* is no easy task, because it requires a purity the Matsigenka readily acknowledge as nearly impossible to achieve. Arafina, a middle-aged Matsigenka woman, told me about the *Saankarite:*

> I would die if I came close to a *Saankarite.* We can't go near them because now we are contaminated. For example, I wear sandals, Mestizo clothes and speak Spanish. We eat onions; things that white people eat. I have a radio. I dance. The *Saankarite* live a happy life there. When they see me, they think I stink. They see me but I don't see them. They don't know death, only happiness. Where they live, it's all clean everywhere. We think they live up on high areas, where it looks as though it's just been swept.

However, when I probed, Arafina said that people in isolated communities untouched by white foreigners were no closer to the *Saankarite.* Other kinds of indecency are believed to taint the more isolated Matsigenka communities: "A mother-in-law can live with her son, and that is forbidden. I've heard of places where they live with their own sons as husbands." The *Saankarite* seem to function as remote, idealized, and stern role models for cultural values that the Matsigenka strive for yet fail to fully embody in their lives on earth. However, the question of whether special people can have access to the heavenly world of the *Saankarite* depends upon prevailing moral assessments of those with supernatural powers. Good spirit contact, or any direct influence of these good forces, seems entirely lacking. This is in contrast to vengeful spirits and sorcery, the effects of which are omnipresent for the Matsigenka. In some way, perhaps, the world of the good spirits is like a paradise lost to mere mortals and in that way similar to the Garden of Eden of Christian cosmology. Death, on the other hand, appears to offer no particular redemptive value to the Matsigenka, as if the impurities and moral failures of the dead inevitably visit the living, to further entrench widespread fear of death and uncertainty about the ill will of others, both the living and the dead.

Being Well and Living a Good Life among the Matsigenka

During open-ended interviews, I asked Matsigenka men and women, young and old, questions such as, "What kinds of things give you happiness, satisfaction, and enjoyment in your life? What sort of experiences bring unhappiness and suffering into your life? How does your present situation compare to the past, and in turn, what is your envisioned future like?" I wanted to understand the goals that people had for themselves and their families in order to contextualize what people were striving for and to determine how satisfied they felt about their present circumstances. My intent was to pose questions that would elicit the Matsigenka's ideal life course in the present and the imagined future.

These questions, which I considered straightforward enough, were quite the contrary for the Matsigenka. While growing up in Chile and in the US, I learned to assess my own personal well-being and satisfaction throughout my life as a matter of course. When I have asked Americans questions such as, "What is well-being to you? What makes you happy? What gives your life meaning? What sort of experiences give you satisfaction?" people might ponder for a moment but quickly give an answer, usually citing health-related ideologies, personal activities (such as going to the gym, running, getting massages, or taking baths), work-related activities, personal relationships, family, and wealth as foundations of well-being (Izquierdo and Paugh 2003). The same questions when asked of the Matsigenka elicited long blank stares. When I probed further and the longer I stayed, I discovered that Matsigenka concepts of happiness and well-being were, by and large, about providing for their families; improving their skills in order to become better hunters, fishermen, and weavers; and maintaining harmonious social relationships. Personal goals or personal pleasurable activities seemed inconceivable, or in any case absent from a discourse that would allow for free-flowing conversation.

When I insisted on getting their views on strictly personal satisfaction, people mentioned playing soccer, weaving, and making *owiroki* (manioc beer) as pleasurable activities. For example, Ramon, a twenty-six-year-old Matsigenka, told me that happiness for him was "to plant in my garden, to support my family by fishing and hunting." Carlos, a thirty-eight-year-old man, said, "I am happy if my house is clean and I have clothes for my children." Most people mentioned very specific needs such as these, which would enhance a sense of satisfaction for themselves and their families. Ultimately, having a sense of well-being had less to do strictly with biological health and more to do with the balance people sought to maintain with their physical and spiritual environment, families, and community in their daily lives.

The Matsigenka do not formulate a clear distinction in their everyday practices between illnesses and states that affect the body, the mind, or their society: emotional, social, and physical well-being are all integral parts of what constitutes a healthy life (Izquierdo 2001; Shepard 1999). The themes I discuss consist of interrelated issues mainly about keeping harmonious interpersonal relations, keeping body and society free of illness, and traditional views of productivity and happiness.

Among the Matsigenka, one's responsibility and respect for family, and the maintenance of nurturing relationships of support are central for achieving well-being. Their immediate and extended families offer the support necessary to enhance well-being. The Matsigenka believe that if they serve their families and follow a strict code of behavior informed by shared cultural values, as evidenced in personal sacrifices in the everyday sharing of food and labor, then well-being will result. In adulthood, the Matsigenka strive to be good providers for their families, which includes being skillful and hardworking (hunters, fishermen, weavers), and maintaining clean bodies and clean households. One must cultivate good family relations by being social, by visiting and sharing (O. Johnson 1978). An important condition for facilitating social relationships lies in keeping a peaceful environment. This is necessary so that each individual can practice self-discipline and control his or her emotions, specifically aggressive emotions, which can lead to conflict and violence. This way they benefit the group as a whole. The Matsigenka will readily sacrifice their own personal goals or stifle their own feelings for the sake of appeasing family and community members.

The formation of communities brought new social obligations and new social order, all of which have resulted in increased conflict, within the family and among community members. Initially (after the formation of the communities), members of other indigenous groups such as Ashaninca and Piro were the chief sources of sorcery accusations. In time however, the Matsigenka began accusing other Matsigenka from distant communities of being sorcerers (*matsikanari*). More recently, sorcery accusations have begun to occur within Matsigenka communities and even within families. Amalia, a twenty-eight-year-old woman, recounted the following events related to illnesses and the influence of outsiders in the Kamisea region:

> This year there are lots of illnesses. I spent lots of time inside my house and didn't go to my garden. More illnesses are coming because Kashiriari [a Shell gas plant in 1998] has gas and the air brings it to us. This year we

will not be happy. Suddenly we won't live anymore. So many people are dying. Before, we lived in peace. Before, we didn't have "*la compañía*" (oil companies). Also their helicopter noise is bothersome. They spill gas and the air then comes here with a bad smell. Sometimes their workers come to Kamisea and get drunk.

Although Amalia does not refer to the distant past, she still has memories of a more peaceful life in Kamisea; she feels strong links between oil companies and noise, pollution, death, and disease. For these disturbances, and particularly new illnesses, she blames outsiders and the oil companies. Ultimately, this translates into a pervasive fear of external forces threatening health and well-being within the community. For Amalia, being happy and at peace were no longer easily achieved because of the constant threat of new and strange illnesses against which she felt powerless. She felt a general deterioration of family values among the younger generations.

Carmelo is a lively and charismatic fifty-year-old Matsigenka man who seeks to hold on to his traditional beliefs and practices but feels pressured by outsiders to give up important Matsigenka values. Carmelo told me of having to conceal his shamanic training and eventually give it up because of missionary pressure. He also described to me the negative influence of schoolteachers on Matsigenka children in eroding community values of goodness: obedience, hard work, collaboration, trust, and sharing—all basic premises for living a good life. According to Carmelo:

> Children used to be obedient to their elders. Even when boys were young, they had their gardens. They weren't lazy like they are now. Now, people don't even want to collaborate in community work. Most important of all, they do not know what it means to share. Young men don't want to learn how to use a bow and arrow properly. They think they will be able to buy shotguns.

The Matsigenka also express confusion regarding their cultural and religious identity in particular, due to missionary Christianization and education. While missionaries and school officials believed formal education to be the answer for the Matsigenka, education was formulated by these outsiders to encapsulate their own values about family size, work, and lifestyle. As Carmelo adds:

> When the missionaries came, they told us "now you will repent before God." I had no idea how to repent, so I just pretended to ask for forgiveness. They told us that now that we were with God, we shouldn't drink *owiroki* or play drums or use our medicinal plants. They told us not to sing. They said: "Your songs are for the devil."

Carmelo's thoughts resonate with views of many other men and women in Kamisea, who see the corrosive effects of outsiders imparting a pervasive sense of shame in the Matsigenka people. The Matsigenka have traditionally had spiritual, emotional, and physical ideas about themselves that contrasted sharply with mainstream Peruvian and missionary notions of identity, especially in terms of conflicting identifications that result from new forms of religion and education.

Both men and women emphasized behavior that contributed to peaceful living, like curbing anger and encouraging autonomy. Men like Carmelo and Alberto spoke of tradition; respect; family support; the importance of sharing and curbing impulses such as fighting, jealousy, or stinginess; and the importance of providing well for the family—all fundamental elements necessary for achieving some degree of well-being. A main concern for both men and women is their ability to be productive and contribute to their households through productive labor.

At a broader social level, societal stress is indexed by an overwhelming increase in sorcery accusations, leading to extreme personal and collective fear, increases in domestic violence, and a pervasive fear of the future. Interestingly, previous researchers working among the Matsigenka of Kamisea, Camaná, and Shimaa during the 1970s and 1980s (O. Johnson 1978; Strongin 1982; Baksh 1984; A. Johnson 2003) concluded that sorcery hardly existed a generation ago. Although Baksh mentions some incidents of sorcery, such cases were mostly associated with a new schoolteacher in the community; Baksh notes that for the Camaná community, "witchcraft has not assumed a role of social control through fear" (1984, 393). Sorcery and witchcraft accusation are absent from Strongin's description of Matsigenka cosmology and illness etiology and diagnosis for the population of Kamisea (1982). The Johnsons in the 1970s found that, although the Matsigenka of Shimaa believed that sorcerers did exist, they did not refer to sorcery as an explanation of illnesses and misfortune. Rather, they explained such suffering as the result of encounters with various forest spirits who inhabited the forest and rock outcrops (A. Johnson 2003; O. Johnson 1978).

The Matsigenka today are terrified of being hexed. They explain the rise in sorcery in terms of stress arising from permanent settlement and untrustworthy outsiders. With settlement came more outsiders and they, in turn, brought increased competition for resources leading to envious feelings (especially relating to Western goods) (Izquierdo and Johnson 2007; Izquierdo et al. 2008), and new and frightening diseases for which they say there are no local cures, such as influenza, measles, and chicken pox. With sorcery accusations on the rise, Kamisea took preventive measures, which involved isolating the community from other Matsigenka communities. Kamisea used to enjoy celebrations (such as the community's anniversary or Peru's independence), where Kamisea would invite other communities for several days of soccer and food. However, in 1998, it was decided that Kamisea would celebrate only among themselves this time. This, they argued in a public meeting, would minimize the risk of anyone being hexed.

Domestic violence was also virtually absent in previous ethnographies and personal accounts of the past. These historical accounts tell of an environment permeated by deep respect for one another and the balance that a clear division of labor brings to a family-level society, where different family members' contributions are essential for survival and harmony. This is important in that along with oil company activity comes a cash economy. The consumption of certain goods may entirely displace the contribution of family members, and especially women's contributions. For example manioc beer (*owiroki* or *masato*) is fundamental to the everyday sociality of the Matsigenka. Women are valued as good providers when there is a steady flow of *owiroki* for all family members and visitors. But if *owiroki* is replaced by bottled beer, men no longer need and value women for their capacity and skill in the making of *owiroki*; instead of congregating with immediate kin, they may seek to share beer with visitors, and may return late to their homes, more inebriated than they would be through drinking *owiroki*. In this situation, domestic violence is more likely to occur. Another serious consequence of gas extraction employment is the fact that local communities export male laborers, leaving women and children behind to manage gardens and to subsist on often-inadequate supplies of fish and game.

The Matsigenka have grown increasingly agitated about the chaos and uncertainty that accompany the massive cultural changes they are experiencing. During the course of my fieldwork, many stories circulated in Kamisea predicting the end of the world. Many of these apocalyptic accounts of doom and disaster were linked to Biblical "proof" that the end was near and that the end of their way of life was, in fact, at hand. Monica, a thirty-year-old Matsigenka woman, told me that in other countries gigantic grasshoppers were eating the plants and the people and that these grasshoppers could not be killed: "The wind will bring them here too and we will all die and disappear," she said. Then Luzmila, an older Matsigenka woman, interjected that they had already found a grasshopper in the vicinity of her house but they were able to kill it. She went on to tell us that the grasshoppers will "kill all our food and our people, this is confirmed in the Bible." Soon after, Alberto (a retired Matsigenka school teacher) asked me if I could help him learn English. Why, I asked. He explained that he had heard news from down river that the *"gringos"* were coming to kill anybody who didn't speak English, especially "old useless people like me." He had heard that "the *gringos* would be more tolerant of young women of reproductive age." Anxiety and uncertainty about the future lie at the heart of these thoughts. These fears encapsulate realities of historical memory mixed with present-day realities that pose a serious threat for Matsigenka lifestyles, values, and well-being.

Another level of anxiety and fear is reflected by the Matsigenka feeling of imposed inferiority, being constantly reminded of their need for "development" and the benefits of "progress." It was striking to see the Matsigenka adopt the language of progress, echoing the acculturation sentiments of settlers and visitors from outside. While the benefits of economic "progress" are certainly evident to the Matsigenka, many also recognize the high price they would pay by becoming bedazzled by material culture and their reliance upon it. Certain goods have been welcomed to facilitate their livelihood, such as clothing, tools, machetes, and shotguns. Other luxury items have begun to flood their society as well, including sunglasses and cameras, and these have quickly gained practical importance. At the same time, such items differentiate members of their society into prestige hierarchies that have little connection to the former dynamics of social status. In fact, community-based authority had historically been limited as family members operated autonomously, and little formal leadership structure existed. Now the parallel processes of settlement and development create different markers of social status that are in direct conflict. On the one hand, the official community leaders grant authority to elected officials who devote their efforts to managing and organizing labor for the common good. On the other hand, some Matsigenka are fast becoming wealthier than others, at least in their display of prestige items, and, more often, in the social power they hold due to ownership of prized items such as shotguns, power tools, boats, and generators.

Conclusion

Well-being includes physical, cognitive/emotional, social, historical, and environmental dimensions, but I argue that the cultural context influences the development and expression of all elements of well-being. It is this cultural context that enables us to understand the central paradox discussed in this paper: physical examinations and laboratory tests confirm that Matsigenka physical health has significantly improved during the past twenty to thirty years, but many Matsigenka seem to feel sicker and suffer more than in the past.

The Matsigenka are undergoing extraordinary cultural change. They moved from a scattered family-based social organization to communities that bring in outsiders and outside knowledge. They report that their quality of life has significantly declined, and attribute their sickness and suffering, by and large, to increased sorcery, outsiders and oil company activity. The suffering and vulnerability that the Matsigenka now experience may reflect a broader crisis of identity and survival in the midst of sweeping social and cultural changes brought on by permanent settlement and recent regional development. Health and education agencies believe that education is the answer to most Matsigenka problems, but education is formulated to encapsulate these agencies' own values concerning family size, work, and lifestyle. Formal education is further redefining notions of cultural identity and aspirations for the Matsigenka. The Matsigenka face strong pressure to comply with the demands of economic development and its social and cultural requirements. Their distress and uncertainty over well-being reflects fears and anxieties over the nature of good and evil in the context of cultural integration and sweeping changes in family roles and values. They view these sweeping changes as evidence of cultural deterioration and as a warning that if current trends continue, the Matsigenka will suffer even more in the future.

As I have sought to show, Matsigenka well-being is defined in terms of physical, social, emotional, spiritual, and environmental components. The experience of well-being is described as the ability to be physically strong enough to work, hunt, and fish; care for family members; keep good social relations; and keep malevolent spirits at bay. Among the Matsigenka, one's responsibility and respect for family and the maintenance of nurturing relationships is an essential component of a good life. The pursuit of self-chosen satisfactions or self-promotion is not a virtue that the Matsigenka promote or cultivate.[6] The immediate and extended family offers fundamental support for the Matsigenka, who tend to believe that if they serve their families and follow a strict code of behavior informed by shared cultural values, then happiness and well-being will result.

But according to many Matsigenka, these ideals of peaceful living are now threatened. They report more households experiencing violence between couples; more frequent and intense drinking of *owiroki,* bottled beer, and hard liquor; a deterioration of family discipline; laziness; and more jealousy and envy. At a personal and cultural level, sorcery afflictions perpetuate blame and suspicion regarding the intentions of outsiders and fellow Matsigenka. As a group, the Matsigenka, living in relative isolation with low population density, were able to avoid destruction in the past, but this may not be the case in the future. Clearly, cultural pressures are shadowing Matsigenka feelings of well-being or its lack. As a group, whether they will be able to survive their current situation remains to be seen—fifty years from now will the Matsigenka still exist? I fear that their loss of well-being today may foreshadow the ultimate end of their society tomorrow.

Notes

Funding from several institutions made this research possible: Fulbright IIE; National Science Foundation Dissertation Research Grant (SBR-9707454); the Anthropology Department at UCLA, and the Alfred P. Sloan Foundation (CELF Center at UCLA). I am very thankful to Elinor Ochs, CELF Director, for her continuous support and encouragement. At CELF I also thank my colleagues Tamar Kremer-Sadlik, Johanna Romero, Adrian Meza, and Paul Connor. Tom Weisner I thank for inspiring me on the subject of well-being. And without Gordon Mathews this project would have been impossible. Thank you, Gordon, for your extensive comments on my chapter, and all our interesting conversations throughout the years. Throughout my graduate years and still today I am also very grateful to Gery Ryan for his comments on my work. In Peru, I am especially thankful to the Matsigenka people for their generosity and friendship.

1. An earlier version of this paper was published in *Social Science and Medicine* in 2005.
2. I will not repeat a review of the literature, since the introductory chapter to this volume as well as Thin's and Colby's chapters discuss in detail the history of the study of well-being in anthropology, and the difficulties we encounter in our formulations of what it means to be well for populations and individuals.
3. This community, very much like most other Matsigenka communities in this region, has a total population of 265 people, living in approximately forty households (houses are easily and frequently dismantled and rebuilt).
4. The rubber boom represents the most hostile period of contact between the Matsigenka, the outside world, and other neighboring groups. Matsigenka were frequently the target of slave-raiders, who forced them to work in latex extraction as the demand for rubber to fuel the military activities of other countries and a demand for rubber in the rest of the world increased steadily. Tragically, slave raiding continued even after the rubber trade had ended.
5. In other references to this designation, I spell *Kamisea* with a K as opposed to *Camisea* with a C, because this is how it would be written in the Matsigenka language.

6. I do not use dichotomies such as sociocentric/collectivist versus individualistic/egocentric because I believe that these terms do not capture the complexity of individual agency and social organization.

References

Adelson, Naomi. 2000. *'Being Alive Well'*: *Health and the Politics of Cree Wellbeing*. Toronto: University of Toronto Press.

Baksh, Michael. 1984. "Cultural Ecology and Change of the Machiguenga Indians of the Peruvian Amazon." PhD thesis, University of California, Los Angeles.

Christopher, John C. 1999. "Situating Psychological Well-being: Exploring the Cultural Roots of its Theory and Research." *Journal of Counseling & Development* 77: 141–52.

Diener, Ed. 1996. "Subjective Well-being in Cross-Cultural Perspective." In *Key Issues in Cross-Cultural Psychology*, ed. H. Grad, A. Blanco, and J. Georgas. Lisse, 319–30. Netherlands: Swets & Zeitlinger.

Gade, Daniel W. 1972. "Comercio y Colonización en la Zona de Contacto entre la Sierra y las Tierras Bajas de Valle del Urubamba en el Peru." *Actas y Memorias del XXXIX Congreso Internacional de Americanistas* 4: 207–21. Lima: Instituto de Estudios Peruanos.

Izquierdo, Carolina. 1995. "The Illness Experience: Health Care Choices Among the Mapuche Living in Santiago." MA thesis, University of California, Los Angeles.

———. 2001. "Betwixt and Between: Seeking Cure and Meaning among the Matsigenka of the Peruvian Amazon." PhD thesis, University of California, Los Angeles.

———. 2005. "When 'Health' is not Enough: Societal, Individual and Biomedical Assessments of Well-being among the Matsigenka of the Peruvian Amazon." *Social Science and Medicine* 61: 727–83.

Izquierdo, Carolina and Conerly Casey. 2003. "Global Consumption of Resources: Witchcraft, Pillage and Plunder in Amazonia and Africa." Paper presented at the International Congress for Americanistas in Santiago, Chile.

Izquierdo, Carolina and Allen W. Johnson. 2007. "Desire, Envy and Punishment: A Matsigenka Emotion Schema in Illness Narratives and Folk Stories." *Culture Medicine and Psychiatry* 31 (4): 419–44.

Izquierdo, Carolina, Allen W. Johnson, and Glenn H. Shepard, Jr. 2008. "Revenge, Envy And Cultural Change in an Amazon Society." In *Revenge in Lowland South America*, ed. Stephen Beckerman and Paul Valentine, 162–86. Gainesville: University Press of Florida.

Izquierdo, Carolina and Amy Paugh. 2003. "Defining and Modeling "Health": Discourses and Practices among Families in Los Angeles." Working Paper Series #10, Sloan Center, UCLA.

Izquierdo, Carolina and Glenn H. Shepard, Jr. 2003. "Matsigenka." *Encyclopedia of Medical Anthropology: Health and Illness in the World's Cultures*. In *Human*

Relations Area Files (HRAF), 823–32. Yale University, ed. Carol R. Ember and Melvin Ember.

Johnson, Allen W. 2003. *Families of the Forest: The Matsigenka Indians of Peruvian Amazon.* Berkeley: University of California Press.

Johnson, Orna R. 1978. "Interpersonal Relations and Domestic Authority among the Machiguenga of the Peruvian Amazon." PhD thesis, Columbia University.

Shepard, Glenn H. Jr. 1999. "Pharmacognosy and the Senses in Two Amazonian Societies." PhD thesis, University of California, Berkeley.

Soto, Julio C. 1982. "Ecología de la Salud en Comunidades Nativas de la Amazonía Peruana." *Amazonía Peruana* 3: 13–26.

Strongin, Jonathan D. 1982. "Machiguenga, Medicine, and Missionaries: The Introduction of Western Health Aids among a Native Population of Southeastern Peru." PhD thesis, Columbia University.

Weiseke, Neva M. 1968. *A Medical Survey of Two Machiguenga Villages.* Beni, Bolovia: Summer Institute of Linguistics.

4

Embodied Selves and Social Selves
Aboriginal Well-Being in Rural New South Wales, Australia
Daniela Heil

Introduction

What does it mean for Australian Aboriginal people to experience well-being and to understand themselves through their conceptions of well-being? Drawing on my ethnography of the small all-Aboriginal village of Murrin Bridge in rural central-western New South Wales, this chapter illustrates ways in which these Aboriginal people understand well-being in response to the quality of their relations with significant, mostly kin-related others. The dominant focus in the neocolonial Australian nation-state, in which indigenous Australians make up 2.4 percent of the national population, is on the well-being of people as individuals—what others and I have termed "embodied selves" (see Moore 1994; Becker 1995; Heil 2003), encompassing the physical and mental state of individuals, their individual bodies and experiences. While Aboriginal people negotiate and respond to this individualistic conception of well-being, they themselves understand and refer to "being well" (the expression they use when paraphrasing what we gloss as "well-being") in relational terms, as an outcome of one's capacity to make and meet the demands and obligations that constitute and reconstitute self-other relationships.

It is common that references to Aboriginal well-being, by Aboriginal people themselves as well as by social and medical scientists, remain oriented to the model of embodied selves. I argue here that this cannot adequately account for Aboriginal people's culturally distinctive ways of prioritizing their *social* selves in their everyday lives. When references to a person's well-being are made, at Murrin Bridge as well as in Aboriginal contexts in other places, it is usually in reference to the well-being of others and rarely to the speaker's own self. At Murrin Bridge, people refer to those who privilege and are preoccupied with their individual selves as "being selfish," "not considering others," and someone who is "not one of us." In order to acknowledge this culturally distinctive understanding of well-being, I argue that a shift is required, from Western conceptualizations of "embodied selves" to Aboriginal understandings of "social selves."

Approaches to "Well-Being"

In order to better understand Murrin Bridge conceptions of well-being in their distinctiveness, I will start with an overview of approaches that have been used to illustrate Western models of well-being across various disciplines. A great number of these emphasize individual psychology (e.g., Diener 1984; Larsen et al. 1985; Nagpal and Sell 1985; Sell and Nagpal 1992; Diener and Suh 2000a; Diener and Suh 2000b) and physical health (e.g., Buunk and Gibbons 1997; Eckersley et al. 2001), conceptualizing the individual as an embodied self with an individualized physical and mental state. Efforts have been made to quantify these studies and to work out reliable instruments for assessing positive and negative indicators, for which Diener (1984; see also Diener and Fujita 1997) as well as Larsen et al. (1985) have provided extensive reviews. Diener and Suh (2000b) also address the study of subjective well-being in a comparative, cross-cultural sense. Emphasizing the need to be able to assess sets of values that characterize a society according to its internal cultural standards, they assign a democratic component to subjective well-being by referring to

> the idea that how each person thinks and feels about his or her life is important. It is not just the opinion of a power elite, or an intellectual class, or psychologists who are experts on "mental health" but through the standards and values chosen by the person herself that societies are evaluated (Diener and Suh 2000b, 4).

However, while this statement highlights differences in each individual, from an anthropological perspective, it is apparent that the authors nevertheless present these subjective understandings of well-being as constant over time, referring to them as personality traits. As we will see in this chapter and its exploring of Aboriginal "social selves," this is not necessarily the case.

Another approach to well-being has been formulated by the World Health Organization (WHO), in linking the notions of health and well-being. This WHO statement situates health within broader, ostensibly more culturally sensitive and appropriate contexts. It refers to health as "not merely the absence of disease [or infirmity], but a state of complete physical, mental, spiritual and social well-being" (1948). This statement is of value in that it broadens the spectrum of health by referring to well-being and, for instance, allows for the inclusion of economic concerns as well (for instance, Frey and Stutzer 2002); however, like the statement in the preceding paragraph, it adopts the individualizing paradigm inherent in Western approaches to health. The understanding taken from health debates and transferred to seemingly more broadly oriented understandings of well-being is the concept of an embodied self and the individual's understandings of what it means to be healthy and well.

Well-being and health are not the same thing. Let me recall a distinction emphasized by Buchanan (2000, 106), who argues that the approach developed by Aristotle is a useful starting point. Aristotle referred to health by stressing biological functioning and referred to well-being (Buchanan's translation of Aristotle's *eudaimonia*) as "happiness," "flourishing," "blessedness," and "prosperity." Although there are different interpretations of *eudaimonia,* the crucial point is that well-being is considered to be the ultimate good, the objective and final goal of all human activity guided by reason. Thus, it is categorically distinct from "natural goods" (also referred to as "instrumental goods") such as health or wealth (Buchanan 2000, 106). In Aristotle's view, health and wealth were instrumental because they were sought not for their own sake but because they supplied a means to bring about some other desired state. As instrumental goods, Aristotle thought that their pursuit could sometimes be harmful, materially and morally, as when individuals place a higher value on pursuing wealth or health than on living an honorable life. In contrast to this, Aristotle considered well-being to be the highest goal of human activity, that which is sought for its own purpose, something towards which all intentional, reasoned practices should ultimately be directed. What this tells us is that well-being is complete in itself and not sought for the purpose of attaining some other end. This model clearly invites us to draw a methodological line, separating the concept of health from that of well-being.

The studies referred to above, in exploring well-being, have often failed to recognize the inherent limitations and individualizing viewpoints that so often derive from Western health-oriented frameworks. Anthropologists, on the other hand, such as Anderson (1999) and Povinelli (1991), as well as Adelson (2000, 1998) and the contributors to this volume, have explored well-being from the perspective of other cultural worlds, avoiding a reiteration of Western ideas of what well-being ought to be.

Murrin Bridge is a prime example of such an "other cultural world." Local Aboriginal people can understand the English term *well-being* but they do not use it much. However, when asked how they "live well," which social practices they like to engage in, what they aim for in their lives, what they value most, or what they consider well-being to be, they usually give answers that can be summarized as "the family being well." Alternatives to this response are "having enough money for the children" or "to be able to enjoy oneself." Other responses are "to get on the grog [drink alcohol] with relatives," "to have enough money for the family," "to have drinks with others at the local pub," or "playing the poker machine with your relatives." As this paper will show, these responses highlight the importance of engagement in social practice for Murrin Bridge people. What are the values that constitute such practices and what do they mean for Murrin Bridge people's "well-being"?

Murrin Bridge: Location and People

The homogenizing term *Aboriginal* camouflages variations of history and cultural practice throughout Australia. While there are pan-Aboriginal commonalities in cultural expression that allow for some generalization, my study is specific to rural New South Wales, part of "settled" Australia, where Aboriginal people have had two hundred years of direct encounter with and control by Anglo-Australian pastoralists, mission managers, and government. Murrin Bridge is 420 miles west-northwest of Sydney, located on the Lachlan River in the central-western district of New South Wales. The latter is the Australian state where Aboriginal people first encountered European occupation and where the struggles with Anglo-Australian influences have their longest history. Aboriginal peoples of New South Wales have dealt with intercultural negotiations as part of their everyday life since 1788 in the east, and about 1850 in the far west of the state. They do not move within domains that are clearly demarcated from the non-Aboriginal world (see Peterson 2000); their lives are intricately enmeshed with that world. This is the case even for an all-Aboriginal settlement such as Murrin Bridge. It was founded as an Aboriginal "station" (a government-managed reserve) in 1949 when the New South Wales government resettled residents from the semiarid areas to the west (for the second time) in order to better implement its policy of assimilation. Local Aboriginal people refer to the station as "the Mission," a widely used term dating from the time when a small number of settlements were run by Christian missionaries. Non-Aboriginal

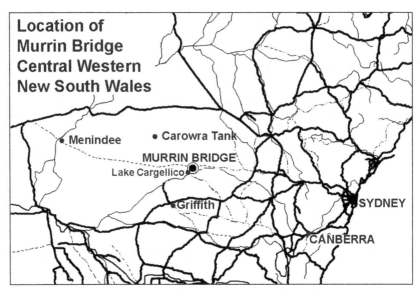

Figure 4.1 Location of Murrin Bridge, Central Western New South Wales

people in the area now frequently use the term in a derogatory way, to devalue the settlement and its people.

Murrin Bridge is located in the far northwestern corner of the country once occupied by speakers of the Wiradjuri language. Today, Aboriginal language areas are recognized as political territories, but the languages are no longer spoken in this region and English, or its variant, Aboriginal English, is the language every Murrin Bridge resident speaks. Wiradjuri country starts west of the Blue Mountains and encompasses a vast regional network of localized kin-based groups spreading across approximately fifty thousand square miles of grasslands, slopes and plains, and rivers and creeks. The majority of Murrin Bridge residents today are people of Ngiyampaa-speaking origin, with a few Paakantji as well, from western New South Wales. This mix is an outcome of government resettlements of Ngiyampaa people in the first half of the twentieth century, first west and then back east. Murrin Bridge residents continue to identify with and trace their ancestry to the semiarid plains of Wangaaypuwan country, between the Lachlan and Darling Rivers. Only a few older people have a working knowledge of the Ngiyampaa language. Apart from a small lexicon of Ngiyampaa words that Wiradjuri people or non-Aboriginal teachers teach the children at the Murrin Bridge preschool, no attempt is made by locals to "keep the lingo," as they say. Since the mid-1990s, the community's population has fluctuated between 135 and 150 people. Most live in the community's thirty-one conventional-style brick houses, with a few older fiberboard houses present as well.

More relatives, kin who have moved away from "the Mission," live "in town," which refers to Lake Cargellico, ten miles south. "Town" represents a broader social and cultural environment, in which responding to social demands and obligations is less intense. The total "town" population comprises over twelve hundred people. Murrin Bridge people might move into town to relieve their boredom (Macdonald and Heil 2008; see also Musharbash 2007), to avoid conflict, or to get away from the intensity of the small community context where "everybody knows everybody's business." At Murrin Bridge, "exchanging the latest goss [gossip]", "having yarns," and "having a cuppa" with others is an essential part of everyday life. Most Murrin Bridge people are closely related, and kin-relatedness directs most social interaction.

Since the establishment of Murrin Bridge in 1949, Aboriginal and non-Aboriginal life worlds have been inextricably intertwined, and continuously negotiated and renegotiated in the community. During the first two decades after the Mission's establishment, the residential managers and schoolteachers applied the government policy of assimilation, promoting the idea that Aboriginal people would undergo non-Aboriginal instructions and then take their place in mainstream Australian society. Until 1967, indigenous affairs in New South Wales had been exclusively a state responsibility. With the passing of a referendum in 1967, indigenous Australians received the right to vote, and the Commonwealth government took on the administration of Aboriginal affairs and legislating on Aboriginal issues. Indigenous Australians became collaterally a federal responsibility. In 1971, the federal Labor Party started to represent itself as the party actively committed to Australian Aborigines and their struggle for land rights, adopting a policy of "self-determination," the idea of which was to enable Aboriginal people to take responsibility for their own affairs. When "self-determination" became Labor's policy, the Liberal Party's response was to call for "self-management," suggesting that Aboriginal people should not only be responsible for their future development but that they should also be held accountable for any success or failure of such development.

Shortly after the 1967 referendum, Murrin Bridge was provided with its own state health service, with the majority of the people working there being non-Aboriginal, or Aboriginal people from other communities who encountered difficulties in finding acceptance in the community because of being nonlocals. Government policies have had a huge impact on Aboriginal peoples' conventional hunter-gatherer practices and have turned Aboriginal people's lives sedentary. The government policies implemented since the early 1970s have failed to alleviate the problem of insufficient work for indigenous Australians, their dependency on welfare payments, and their personal despair.

Today, Murrin Bridge people's and other Australian Aboriginal experiences reflect a volatile world. Anthropologist Jeremy Beckett (1978, 1988, 1993) pioneered study in this region of central-western New South Wales from the 1950s on, in work that challenged the more popular study of the exotic and the traditional in Australian Aboriginal research. More recently, anthropologists have examined increasing Aboriginal activism, and the demand by Aboriginal peoples for civil rights and land rights in their aspirations for justice, equality, and citizenship (see, for instance, Macdonald 2004, 1988 on land rights; and Cowlishaw 1988, and Cowlishaw and Morris 1997 on racist incidents). Over the five-and-a-half decades since the establishment of their community, Murrin Bridge people have been dealing with social change, and negotiating and adapting to it, in their own distinctive ways. Their understandings, including those of "being well," emerge from their often conflicting and difficult, adaptive and counter-adaptive history, both reflecting and creating their cultural distinctiveness within mainstream Australian society.

By illustrating what Murrin Bridge people value in being well and living well, I seek to avoid the tendency to demarcate separate Aboriginal/non-Aboriginal domains as if their distinctive dynamics simply meet head-on from time to time. Contemporary anthropological studies in Australia now deal more sensitively with the ways in which Aboriginal peoples address change in their lives, vis-à-vis mainstream Australian society (for instance, Robinson 1997; Macdonald 2001; Peterson and Taylor 2003; Austin-Broos 2003b). These studies contribute to an understanding of cultural practice and well-being as continuous, dynamic products of Murrin Bridge people's interactions with each other and with the multifaceted broader environment. Understandings of well-being in Murrin Bridge emerge from the dynamic cultural world within which Murrin Bridge people negotiate their intercultural lives and culturally distinctive identities within the Australian nation-state.

My Own Involvement with Murrin Bridge

I began field work in Murrin Bridge in 1999, living in the community for eighteen months. I continue to visit, maintaining my commitment to local people and friends, and catching up on the latest happenings, events, and stories. During my field research, I lived in three differ-

ent homes, at different ends of "the Mission," each for three months or
longer. While this was not planned in advance, I can see in retrospect
how this broadened my experience of communal life. It gave me the opportunity to become more familiar with different people and their particular kin-groupings' perspectives on local and other issues. I was able
to discern the various social groupings and their networks of kin and
fellow workers. Being with different people, their stories, understandings, beliefs, and comments helped my understanding of community
politics and frictions over time. Each of my Aboriginal "relatives," as
they became from our joint residence, was of a different generation and
a member of a different constellation of social networks. These people
and their close kin are nodes from whom I have continued to gather
a comprehensive and extensive understanding of what it means to be
well at Murrin Bridge.

The initial focus of my research was Aboriginal understandings of
diabetes. However, this focus changed when I began to realize that diabetes and its long-term management—despite its prevalence—was of
no particular interest to local Aboriginal people. People do know that
it is a problem. However, despite this, they will make comments such
as, "I do not consider it a number one priority in my life," or "it doesn't
worry me." I wanted to know what they meant by such statements;
their answers to my questions directed me to people's paths through
life. I began to ask, "What does it mean to you 'to be well'? Why is
it more important to look after your relatives than to look after yourself and your body? What does it mean to be 'one of us'?" I started to
examine the language and practice that would lead me to understand
Aboriginal approaches to well-being.

Over time, having been treated as "one of us" by Murrin Bridge people, I have come to understand that being well derives from the ways
in which people prioritize self-other relationships, which illustrates the
meanings of "being one of us." Local Aboriginal people accepted me as
a participant in their communal life and practice and taught me their
ways of being in the world. They have always been prepared to give me
feedback on my understandings and analyses of their lives and practices, and have trusted me to use their stories, as in this chapter. Murrin Bridge people consider respect and accountability as being central
to relationships, whether to kin, to non-kin such as myself, and even
within the broader Australian society. These relationships are not constituted overnight, but derive from interactions and familiarity, built up
over time. Relationships are not taken for granted and are continuously
reconstituted and renewed through one's presence in the social and engagement in socialities. Local Aboriginal people who leave communal

life because they may be sick in a hospital or because they just "went off for a while" have to reconstitute their social credentials through meaningful participation when they return. As many Murrin Bridge people explain, "you have to be on the ball and stay on the ball to be one of us." What they mean is that to be valued and responded to as "one of us," and to have the right to make demands on others, one has to continuously be a responsible and responsive participant in local kin-based affairs. One is expected to share stories and gossip, to look after others, and to be willing to be looked after.

My presence over many months in Murrin Bridge enabled me to become a member of a "mob," which is how Aboriginal people refer to significant others, most usually a reference to kin. Weiner (1995, 6) argues that the anthropologist's long-term involvement in people's lives "implies more than recording people's stories: it means being entailed in and by their lives and bearing the inevitable consequences of having the effects of those lives impinge upon one's own." This reflects my own understanding of the methodology I have adopted in undertaking research in Aboriginal Australia.

Aboriginal Well-Being at Murrin Bridge

Murrin Bridge Life and Practice

To explore the cultural understandings of Aboriginal well-being and how these differ from non-Aboriginal understandings, I return to Buchanan's approach to well-being as a process of becoming, realized through living well and engaging in social practices that embody the values people wish to bring into being. So my question is, what constitutes Murrin Bridge life and practice, and how do the social practices people engage in contribute to local Aboriginal people's understandings of well-being? By practice, I refer to Bourdieu's practical logic of everyday action as well as the objective structures within which these actions take place. Each person who participates in social practice is a producer and reproducer of objective meaning. At the same time, each person's activities are "the product of a *modus operandi* of which [that person] is not the producer" (Bourdieu 1977, 79; see also Burkitt 1991). Practice "unfolds in time" (Bourdieu 1990, 81), and has a temporal dimension—a particular, culturally determined rhythm, tempo, and directionality (see Heil and Macdonald 2008) that is constitutive of its meanings.

The shaping of Murrin Bridge practice stems largely from the demands of kin-relatedness, and the integration of these relations into leisure time and work—although these are not distinctions made by Murrin Bridge people themselves. When using the expression "work," Murrin Bridge people primarily refer to attending the Lake Cargellico vocational training college (known as TAFE: T-raining A-nd F-urther E-ducation), which runs a variety of educational courses, based on a weekly payment for attending, and working on the Community Development Employment Project, known as CDEP, which is the project in which most Murrin Bridge residents participate. CDEP combines welfare receipt with a work program (known among non-Aboriginal people as "working for the dole"). Initiated and implemented by the federal government, its central purpose is for Aboriginal people to earn unemployment entitlements by working on community projects and, in this way, to do something for their own living space. The government's rhetoric suggests that CDEP work will establish personal initiative and activity and encourage the taking on of responsibility. The perspective of most Murrin Bridge people is that CDEP work enables you "to look after your family, other relations, and yourself." What is characteristic of this comment, applying to Murrin Bridge people generally, is that relatives are usually mentioned prior to oneself. This is a moral orientation supported by most people at Murrin Bridge: "You'll be right as long as you take care of your family." "Family" refers not only to immediate kin but also to a wide range of people in a kin-defined network who may or may not be co-resident.

Apart from the majority of Murrin Bridge people working on CDEP or going to TAFE, there are currently four Murrin Bridge people who work and who are referred to by kin as having "a proper job." Often, such commentators may add a negative comment to this, such as "they think they're better than we are," reflecting the idea that these people hold permanent jobs that provide a regular income. One Murrin Bridge resident has been a truck driver for over twenty-five years, another works as a liaison officer at the hospital in town, and another has held the position of police liaison officer for over seven years. This means that their incomes are higher than the majority of Murrin Bridge "workers." For the latter, the key objective of work-related practices is "to have money in your pocket": money opens up all kinds of social opportunities. However, unemployment is high in this region, in particular for Aboriginal people, and the main source of income, apart from TAFE and CDEP money, is social security, including aged and single parent pensions, child allowances, and unemployment benefits.

The activities linked to the availability of financial resources occur in conjunction with paydays, in some cases weekly, in others fortnightly. "Pay day" is the local term for the day on which CDEP money, TAFE

money, and pension and social security payments are received. On paydays, Murrin Bridge people usually leave early to get into town. People
who have cars drive, others may get a ride with a relative, and others
again may decide to walk to the main road, about half a mile from the
Mission, to get a lift with someone "who might be heading to town."
As soon as they are in town, people queue at one of the two banks to
withdraw their money. Then they will go to buy groceries, pay bills (for
instance, rent, electricity, telephone, paying off the television), and, if required, respond to kin who might have claims because they have been
"good to you." As soon as "the fridge is full, and a bill or two" have
been paid, Aboriginal people at the Mission and in town start enjoying
themselves. The local expression "enjoying yourself" refers to gather-
ings that encourage interacting with others, such as playing cards, or
buying cigarettes and cartons of beer to share with one's mob. Someone
might fill up a car with gasoline to visit relatives in town or to play the
poker machine at one of the local pubs. The use of illicit drugs started in
the mid-1980s and has increased continuously since. It now forms part
of "enjoying yourself" as well. In the words of one Murrin Bridge elder,
the consumption of drugs has introduced "selfishness, and that keeps
destroying our culture and its values." What she means is that drug us-
ers position their personal needs first. She continues, "They don't care
about their mothers and fathers and other rellies [relatives] any more,
they just care about themselves. That's whitefella [non-Aboriginal] way,
but that's not our way." There is a wealth of meaning in this statement:
it refers to the destruction of cultural values through the prioritizing of
oneself over social obligations and responsibilities; it also reveals the
ongoing challenges Aboriginal people confront in negotiating Western
ideals of what it means to be a person. The statement implies that the
"whitefella way" encourages competitiveness, privileges the embodied
self, and positions oneself above obligations to kin.

A distinctive Aboriginal practice at Murrin Bridge and in other parts
of the continent is *demand sharing* (see Macdonald 2000 for southeastern
Australia; Peterson 1997, 1993 for northern Australia). Demand sharing describes the practice of sharing as a social obligation. Kin have
a right to demand and receive available resources that others possess, and likewise have an obligation to share what they have. Things
"shared" (given in response to a demand) may include cash, food,
gasoline, cigarettes, and, in winter, wood. Demand sharing recognizes
"social obligations on the part of those who control resources rather
than indebtedness on the part of those who receive them" (Macdonald
2000, 91). It is a system that continually constitutes and reconstitutes relatedness between people, emphasizing face-to-face engagement, and

testing social responsibilities and obligations defined by kin-related-ness. Demand sharing supports the working of the kin-related net-work. As an outcome of these interactive values, the well-being of one's mob depends on the ways in which each member responds to social demands by fulfilling social obligations. Despite having an interactive emphasis, demand sharing creates an imbalance because it does not require reciprocity. It is based on one's rights as kin rather than the obligation to exchange. This sustains the notion that social dynamics are contingent (see Heil and Macdonald 2008), and that Aboriginal ways of sharing neither reflect nor comply with Western understand-ings of reciprocal giving and taking. Demand sharing in Murrin Bridge is a practice transformed from the formerly hunter-gatherer economy (Macdonald 2000; Peterson 1993) which governs the intra-Aboriginal domestic and kin-oriented economy today as well (see also Peterson and Taylor 2003).

An example illustrates the value of demand sharing. Kevin is a Mur-rin Bridge resident in his early fifties, trained as a registered nurse, and "someone who has lived in both worlds," as he puts it. He now earns money by working ten hours per week on CDEP and going to TAFE four mornings per week. During last year's CDEP break over the hot summer, the six weeks from Christmas to the end of January, Kevin expected to live only on his TAFE vacation allowance. TAFE students who intend to continue their training after that break, receive "vaca-tion money," an up-front payment at the beginning of the holidays, expected to cover them financially over the vacation period. Towards the end of each TAFE year, continuing students have to submit a form indicating to the head office that they will be continuing next year and require "vacation money." Last year Kevin was a week late submitting his form. When he eventually managed to fax it to the head office, "the form went missing"; in Kevin's words, "they mucked up my vacation money." For Kevin, this meant that he was without an income until the end of January. Kevin was upset not because he would be unable to pay his bills, but because he was not able to maintain autonomy within his social network of kin-obligation, which requires having access to resources such as cash. He was unable to respond to the demands of others and felt uncomfortable. He had no choice but to make demands on others, making him socially irresponsive over that time. The issue is not that people would not understand and support him, but that he lost his (highly valued) personal autonomy in always being the asker.

In the small community of Murrin Bridge, news travels quickly. Within a day everybody knew that "Kevin is in bad shape," that he would be unable to meet his financial obligation to pay for drinks with his mob, to play cards, and to give cigarettes to relatives on demand. However, according to Kevin, the valued part of his story to me was that "it [demand sharing] always works. Your relatives will always feed you and help you when you go through a difficult patch. You are never on your own, even if you want to be. They never leave you alone." Murrin Bridge people will always receive the support of other members of their kin network; and as long as a person is socially present, she or he is unable to withdraw from the social demands and obligations which constitute, maintain, and reconstitute the self and the socialities in which he or she is engaged over time.

Aboriginal Well-Being

How can we understand Aboriginal well-being, considering that Murrin Bridge people's engagement in social practices reflects their cultural values and prioritizing and, consequently, is a crucial constituent in the process of becoming well (cf. Buchanan 2000)? There are studies focusing on Australian Aboriginal peoples that include a notion of well-being but which have not explored people's culturally distinctive understandings in greater detail (see, for example, Austin-Broos 2003a, 1996; Povinelli 1993, 1991; Robinson 1997; Holmes et al. 2002). Other anthropologists have linked "not being well" to, for instance, low socio-economic status and the marginalization of Aboriginal Australians (for instance, Myers 1986; Macdonald 2000; Peterson and Taylor 2003). These studies provide an important contribution to understanding the enormity of the task Aboriginal peoples may face in negotiating intracultural demands and obligations derived from their former hunter-gatherer economy with their contemporary position within the Australian market economy. Ninety-eight percent of the current Murrin Bridge population depend on government welfare payments, which in effect measure Aboriginal lives by non-Aboriginal living standards, social and cultural understandings, and what is often depicted as desirable norms. This demonstrates disrespect for Aboriginal cultural values and experiences, and creates a continuing disjuncture between Western and indigenous Australian understandings of well-being.

Studies linking Australian Aboriginal health to well-being often emphasize the availability of sewerage, food, water, electricity, housing, and economic independence (for instance, Sykes 1989; Mobbs 1991, 297–302;), using "Aboriginal health" and "Aboriginal well-being" as synonyms without exploring their distinction. Aboriginal medical practitioner and anthropologist Ian Anderson (1999, 65) provides a more nuanced approach, stating that the core elements of Aboriginal understandings of well-being involve "the physical, social, emotional, cultural and spiritual well-being not only of the individual but of the whole community." Well-being, he writes, comprises "people, place and law, and is a whole-of-life view, including the traditional concept of life-death-life as well as the relationship to the land" (Anderson 1999, 65). Although his reference to tradition suggests a static understanding (see Macdonald 2001), Anderson's commentary is useful in that he emphasizes that well-being is not restricted to the individual and his or her material conditions but to the whole community. Anderson's "Aboriginal" approach alerts us to the relationships between people within communal frameworks. He offers, like Aristotle as we earlier saw, a whole-of-life view that embraces understandings of health but is not reduced to them. This is what is encapsulated in Aboriginal experiences of well-being, which move away from the conventional medical focus on individuals as embodied selves, to instead include the social positioning of individuals, their historical experiences, and their being members and participants in a matrix of relationships and social practices.

In my own work, I have explored Aboriginal people's understandings of health and well-being, the distinctiveness of their understandings in relation to non-Aboriginal perspectives, and how these understandings are situated within Aboriginal socialities and health practices (Heil 2003). I have been critical of the fact that, particularly with regard to Aboriginal peoples in "settled" Australia, whose cultural worlds have been drastically changed throughout colonial, postcolonial, and neocolonial history, health and well-being are persistently seen as synonymous, when to Aboriginal people themselves, they are *not* synonymous. This approach has been taken by other anthropologists as well; for instance, David McKnight (2002, 6), exploring social change over a period of thirty years among Aboriginal people on Mornington Island, off the north Queensland coast, argues that non-Aboriginal Australian government officials "act in accordance to what *they* think would be good for the community" (my emphasis) and its Aboriginal population, without taking account of what Aboriginal peoples themselves may think. Kevin, quoted above, commented on the problem of negotiating culturally distinctive understandings in terms of non-Aboriginal/Aboriginal law:

> You have all these Gubbas [whitefellas] who turn up here. They are experts from university, experts on drugs, alcohol, sexual abuse, domestic violence, and so on, and they probably do the best they can. But they don't have the foggiest idea of black people and black communities.

What he means is that limiting the understanding of a problem to "whitefella law" or "whitefella perceptions," such as conventional attitudes to drug use or alcohol consumption, cannot encompass the communal, kin-related, and historical network of relationships that an Aboriginal person is likely to be enmeshed in every day.

What It Means to "Be Well" in Murrin Bridge

At Murrin Bridge, older people are wont to say, "what's mine is yours, and what's yours is mine. It's ours, it's all the same." What they mean is that they do not understand themselves as monads, as solitary individuals, separable from others. And even though they place a high value on autonomy—emphasizing each person's social autonomy as the realization of their responsibility for themselves—it is not independence but an autonomy that is continuously constituted *within* the social, not apart from it. Murrin Bridge people are *social* selves (Burkitt 1991) and they grapple uncomfortably with the demands of Anglo-Australians that they be individual embodied selves, with the ensuing values and moral codes that this entails.

Murrin Bridge life and practice, such as demand sharing and other engagements with one's mob, focus on activities that continuously reaffirm the social. To engage in these activities means to be part of a modus operandi within which each person's social self is affirmed and reconstituted by her or his participating in the ongoing social world and its matrix of relationships. What this means is that such everyday activities as "working on CDEP" or "going to TAFE," will not necessarily produce the individuated values assumed of such participation by the mainstream society. Instead of investing in their own individual economic future, participants in such programs are more likely to share the resulting resources (wages) in social investment in kin-relatedness.

Aboriginal understandings of well-being are the product of this world of social practice. As Murrin Bridge people explain, "it is *being there* that makes you well." What they are referring to is the value they place on social presence and *active* engagement in the social. According to Kelly, another Murrin Bridge resident, "I am well when something is happening around me." Asked whether she was able to experience the same extent of wellness on her own, she responded with a clear "No! On your own, nothing happens, everything is boring!" When I suggested to her that it is "others [in particular, relatives] who make you well," she gave me a big smile and said, "Of course! You know what we're like, you're one of us." What Kelly meant is that responding to kin and social obligations are prerequisites for constituting "being well"—or "well-being," to use the increasingly popular Western phrasing. For Murrin Bridge people, well-being requires one "to be there," meaning that one is able to make the effort required to participate in the social or respond to the approaches of others.

The alternative to being there is *being absent,* which is to be unable to participate in the social. The nonparticipant is not considered by those who are there. When Albert had to spend two weeks away in a Sydney hospital in an intensive care unit because of a life-threatening kidney infection, he experienced a social death. Being at home in Murrin Bridge would have enabled him to engage and participate in social practices with his mob, even if ill. His presence would have enabled him to make and respond to demands. He would have had the opportunity to be responsive or irresponsive to the demands of kin-related others. However, not having had a choice, and being required to be absent, he was not in the position of being able to be well. From a Western perspective on health and well-being, Albert did what he had to do to become well physically: he looked after his embodied self. From Albert's Aboriginal perspective, his absence and "being away from home," as he put it, neglected his matrix of social relationships, put them at risk, and initiated a process that potentially could lead to the destruction of his social self through being forgotten. Consequently, to be absent, though necessary for physical health, impacts very negatively on his well-being.

Kelly's comment and Albert's experience, two examples of many I could cite, demonstrate that Aboriginal people on their own experience a state akin to social death. By not "being there," by withdrawing from the social, Murrin Bridge people put their mob membership and the ongoing reconstitution and affirmation of their personhood at risk. The withdrawal of sociality, for whatever reason, can be terrifying and many will avoid treatment programs that require them to be away from home. While Albert had no choice but to continue his intensive care treatment until getting physically better, he went to great lengths to try and send messages home to alleviate his distress and to ensure his social rehabilitation upon his return. Kevin, as we earlier saw, had for financial reasons no choice but to position himself in a dependency relationship with kin, contradicting the value he and they would normally place on autonomy as a person's responsibility to look after themselves. In doing so, he was accumulating indebtedness that he would have to balance out later on if he was to reestablish a nondependent relationship and regain personal autonomy within relatedness (see also Myers 1986) and other people's respect. For him, relying on his kin network (sisters, nieces, and cousins) was not so much the need for economic and other resources for his *embodied self.* Rather, his primary concern was the continuation of his engagement in the social despite his lack of resources. While he might have been able to access cash away from the community, this would have had a more negative effect on his well-being than the short-term economic dependence on kin that maintained his position within the social.

For Aboriginal people at Murrin Bridge—and perhaps in Aboriginal Australia more generally—being well is inseparable from "being at home" and situated within the social. Being well is a process of self-making through social identification, a sign of the health of a social self-in-the-world, one who is in a proper relationship to kin. Well-being is rooted in cultural norms and values that permeate and define—and yet extend beyond—the individual, her or his physicality and embodied self. Well-being is the result of an ongoing dynamic process that constitutes and reconstitutes the social person and the socialities of which they are part and to which they contribute. Social health is a dynamic process that is the instrumental good for constituting well-being, which can be paraphrased as "the highest goal of human activity." In this sense, Aboriginal well-being is a social reality, achieved through the engagement of social selves who are able to access the resources (especially cash) through which they negotiate and mediate their selves and socialities. This means that "well-being" is not something that can be understood as a constant. Murrin Bridge people's understandings of well-being, as responses to the quality of one's social engagement, shift with time and place. It depends on each person, and how they perceive and contribute to their social health from one day to the next.

Conclusion

Aboriginal social selves are fundamentally interdependent. Aboriginal people's social participation remains the essence of personhood and, accordingly, this is the essence of what it means for them to be socially valued and hence well. Their embodied experience is not contained within an individual body but within a social one, defined and informed by kin-relatedness and its practices. Practices of well-being are ultimately sanctioned by the degree to which they are able to better locate the embodied self within the nexus of social relatedness. Burkitt's (1991) theory of social selves is a helpful path into the distinctiveness of Aboriginal notions of social selves, resisting as it does the dichotomizing of "individual" and "society." Burkitt argues that, even in "the West," it is social relations that lie behind our conscious awareness of our existence as individuals, and that even "the Western self" is fundamentally social. It is social life that is the source of the individuality of Western modernity, and human beings only develop as individuals—as fulfilled humans—within a social context. What this means is that so-cial relations—not just between Aboriginal people, but between all of us in the world to at least some extent—constitute, reconstitute, and con-tinue to shape the collectivity and its moral order.

From a Western perspective, Aboriginal well-being does not neces-sarily point to a cheerful or healthy individual, nor is it something that necessarily benefits the individual as an embodied self. Rather, the en-tire community is the beneficiary of Aboriginal well-being and, accord-ingly, encompasses each person as well. To experience being well, being there and participating in the social are prerequisites for Aboriginal people, but for non-Aboriginal people, the intensity of this participation can be exhausting. Few try it and thus few understand its constraints and strengths. However, even though non-Aboriginal people are often critical of Aboriginal responses to well-being that seem to them to be contradictory, for the Aboriginal person, being well-integrated socially offers more than well-being: it also offers a means of making sense of the profoundly demanding and often disturbing negotiations required of interculturally marginalized communities, often living with high levels of stress, and partaking of the politics of dealing with an often discriminatory non-Indigenous "other." Nevertheless, even while intra-Aboriginal engagement seems to be progressively squeezed into smaller and smaller economic, political, and social spaces within the Austra-lian nation-state, Aboriginal people's engagement with nonindigenous practice simultaneously continues to open up spaces for new forms of meaning. The acknowledging of Aboriginal understandings of well-being within mainstream Australian society has the potential to pro-duce both greater awareness of Aboriginal cultural sensitivities and also a critique of taken-for-granted Western conceptions of well-being.

References

Adelson, Naomi. 1998. "Health Beliefs and the Politics of Cree Well-Being." *Health* 2: 5–22.

———. 2000. *'Being Alive Well': Health and the Politics of Cree Well-Being.* Toronto: University of Toronto Press.

Anderson, Ian. 1999. "Aboriginal Well-Being." In *Health in Australia: Sociological Concepts and Issues,* ed. Carol Grbich, 53–73. Sydney: Prentice Hall.

Austin-Broos, Diane J. 1996. "'Two Laws', Ontologies, Histories: Ways of Being Aranda Today." *The Australian Journal of Anthropology* 7: 1–20.

———. 2003a. "Globalisation and the Genesis of Values." *The Australian Journal of Anthropology* 14: 1–18.

———. 2003b. "Places, Practices, and Things: The Articulation of Arrernte Kin-ship with Welfare and Work." *American Ethnologist* 30: 118–35.

Becker, Anne E. 1995. *Body, Self, and Society: The View from Fiji.* Philadelphia: University of Pennsylvania Press.

Beckett, Jeremy R. 1978. "George Dutton's Country: Portrait of an Aboriginal Drover." *Aboriginal History* 2: 2–30.

———. 1988. "The Past in the Present, the Present in the Past: Constructing a National Aboriginality." In *Past and Present: The Construction of Aboriginality*, ed. Jeremy R. Beckett, 191–217. Canberra: Aboriginal Studies Press.

———. 1993. "Walter Newton's History of the World – or Australia." *American Ethnologist* 20: 675–95.

Bourdieu, Pierre. 1977. *Outline of a Theory of Practice.* Cambridge: Cambridge University Press.

———. 1990. *The Logic of Practice.* Stanford, CA: Stanford University Press.

Buchanan, David R. 2000. *An Ethic for Health Promotion: Rethinking the Sources of Human Well-Being.* New York: Oxford University Press.

Burkitt, Ian. 1991. *Social Selves. Theories of the Social Formation of Personality.* London: Sage Publications.

Buunk, Bram P. and Frederick X. Gibbons, eds. 1997. *Health, Coping, and Well-Being: Perspectives from Social Comparison Theory.* London: Lawrence Erlbaum Associates.

Cowlishaw, Gillian. 1988. *Black, White or Brindle: Race in Rural Australia.* Sydney: Cambridge University Press.

Cowlishaw, Gillian and Barry Morris, eds. 1997. *Race Matters: Indigenous Australians and 'Our' Society.* Canberra: Aboriginal Studies Press.

Diener, Ed. 1984. "Subjective Well-Being." *Psychological Bulletin* 95: 542–75.

Diener, Ed and Frank Fujita. 1997. "Social Comparisons and Subjective Well-Being." In *Health, Coping, and Well-Being: Perspectives from Social Comparison Theory,* ed. Bram P. Buunk and Frank X. Gibbons, 329–57. London: Lawrence Erlbaum Associates.

Diener, Ed and Eunkook M. Suh, eds. 2000a. *Culture and Subjective Well-Being.* Cambridge, MA: MIT Press.

Diener, Ed and Eunkook M. Suh. 2000b. "Measuring Subjective Well-Being to Compare the Quality of Life of Cultures." In *Culture and Subjective Well-Being,* ed. Ed Diener and Eunkook M. Suh, 3–12. Cambridge, MA: MIT Press.

Eckersley, Richard, Jane Dixon, and Bob Douglas, eds. 2001. *The Social Origins of Health and Well-Being.* Cambridge: Cambridge University Press.

Frey, Bruno S. and Alois Stutzer. 2002. *Happiness and Economics: How the Economy and Institutions Affect Well-Being.* Princeton, NJ: Princeton University Press.

Heil, Daniela. 2003. "Well-Being and Bodies in Trouble: Situating Health Practices within Australian Aboriginal Socialities." PhD thesis. University of Sydney: Department of Anthropology.

Heil, Daniela and Gaynor Macdonald. 2008. "'Tomorrow Comes When Tomorrow Comes': Managing Aboriginal Health within an Ontology of Life-as-Contingent." *Oceania* 78 (3): 299–319.

Holmes, Wendy, Paul Stewart, Anne Garrow, Ian Anderson, and Lisa Thorpe. 2002. "Researching Aboriginal Health: Experience from a Study of Urban Young People's Health and Well-Being." *Social Science and Medicine* 54: 1267–79.

Larsen, Randy J., Ed Diener, and Robert A. Emmons. 1985. "An Evaluation of Subjective Well-Being Measures." *Social Indicators Research* 17: 1–17.

Macdonald, Gaynor. 1988. "Self-Determination or Control: Aborigines and Land Rights Legislation in New South Wales." *Social Analysis* 24: 34–49.

———. 2000. "Economies and Personhood: Demand Sharing among the Wiradjuri of New South Wales." In *The Social Economy of Sharing: Resource Allocation and Modern Hunter-Gatherers,* ed. G.W. Wenzel, G. Hovelsrud-Broda, and N. Kishigami, 87–111. Osaka, Japan: National Museum of Ethnology.

———. 2001. "Does 'Culture' Have 'History'? Thinking about Continuity and Change in Central New South Wales." *Aboriginal History* 25: 176–99.

———. 2004. *Two Steps Forward, Three Steps Back: A Wiradjuri Land Rights Journey.* Canada Bay, Australia: LhR Press.

Macdonald, Gaynor and Daniela Heil. n.d. "Boredom as Cultural Practice: The Unspoken Dilemma Facing Australian Aboriginal Communities." Manuscript.

McKnight, David. 2002. *From Hunting to Drinking: The Devastating Effects of Alcohol on an Australian Aboriginal Community.* London: Routledge.

Mobbs, Robyn. 1991. "In Sickness and Health: The Sociocultural Context of Aboriginal Well-Being, Illness and Healing." In *The Health of Aboriginal Australia,* ed. Janice Reid and Peggy Trompf, 292–325. Sydney: Harcourt and Brace.

Moore, Henrietta. 1994. "Embodied Selves: Dialogues between Anthropology and Psychoanalysis." In *A Passion for Difference: Essays in Anthropology and Gender,* 28–48. Bloomington: Indiana University Press.

Musharbash, Yasmine. 2007. "Boredom, Time, and Modernity: An Example from Aboriginal Australia." *American Anthropologist* 109: 307–17.

Myers, Fred. 1986. *Pintupi Country, Pintupi Self: Sentiment, Place and Politics among Western Desert Aborigines.* Washington, DC: Smithsonian Institution Press.

Nagpal, Rup and Helmut Sell. 1985. *Subjective Well-Being.* New Delhi: World Health Organization.

Peterson, Nicolas. 1993. "Demand Sharing: Reciprocity and the Pressure for Generosity among Foragers." *American Anthropologist* 95: 860–74.

———. 1997. "Demand Sharing: Sociobiology and the Pressure for Generosity among Foragers?" In *Scholar and Sceptic: Australian Aboriginal Studies in Honour of Les Hiatt,* ed. Francesca Merlan, John Morton, and Alan Rumsey, 171–90. Canberra: Aboriginal Studies Press.

———. 2000. "An Expanding Aboriginal Domain: Mobility and the Initiation Journey." *Oceania* 70 (3): 205–18.

Peterson, Nicolas and John Taylor. 2003. "The Modernising of the Indigenous Domestic Moral Economy." *The Asia Pacific Journal of Anthropology* 4: 105–22.

Povinelli, Elizabeth. 1991. "The Production of Political, Cultural, and Economic Well-Being at the Belyuen Aboriginal Community, Northern Territory of Australia." PhD thesis. Yale University.

———. 1993. *Labor's Lot: The Power, History, and Culture of Aboriginal Action.* Chicago: University of Chicago Press.

Robinson, Gary. 1997. "Trouble Lines: Resistance, Externalization and Individuation." *Social Analysis* 41: 122–54.

Sell, Helmut and Rup Nagpal. 1992. *Assessment of Subjective Well-Being: The Subjective Well-Being Inventory (SUBI)*. New Delhi: World Health Organization.

Sykes, Roberta B. 1989. *Black Majority. An Analysis of 21 Years of Black Australian Experience as Emancipated Australian Citizens*. Hawthorn, Australia: Hudson.

Weiner, James F. 1995. "Anthropologists, Historians and the Secret of Social Knowledge." *Anthropology Today* 2 (5): 3–7.

WHO. 1948. Preamble to the Constitution of the World Health Organization as adopted by the International Health Conference, New York, 19–22 June 1946.

5

THE SHIFTING LANDSCAPE OF CREE WELL-BEING

Naomi Adelson

To understand the cultural meanings of well-being is to understand a society's social, cultural, and political values: values which are, in turn, reflected in the language and practices of well-being. Much as culture is understood as being dynamic, so too are notions of well-being, and those meanings will change over time and with changes to our wider social and political landscapes (cf. Lock and Scheper-Hughes 1990; Mann 2005). In this chapter, I examine the ways in which a particular Aboriginal conceptualization of well-being is at once both grounded in specific land-based beliefs and activities and yet is changing with changing times. Other Canadian studies of First Nations' and Métis' well-being have focused expressly on the balanced interrelationship of spiritual, emotional, physical, and mental soundness as central to well-being. Those works highlight a distinctive Aboriginal concept of well-being through an embodied self that has, not surprisingly, been deeply affected by a history of colonial imposition and constraints. There has been, however, relatively little focus on the more immediate social or political contexts through which people's concepts of a balanced well-being shifts or changes (Bartlett 2004; Wilson 2004).

Here, I present a discussion of well-being as it is articulated by the eastern Cree of Quebec, Canada, that, as for so many other indigenous groups worldwide, begins with an expression of well-being as literally, symbolically, and strategically linked to land. The literal and metaphoric space of eastern Cree well-being is a vast territory that defines nothing less than the history and future of the Cree nation. That landscape, however, has changed over the decades and with it, so too have the Cree people and the ways that well-being is articulated as part of their relationship to that land.

Historical Background

Let me begin with a specific example of that relationship. In a 1985 submission to the United Nations Commission on Human Rights Working

Group on Indigenous Populations, the Grand Council of the Crees began with this statement:

> The Grand Council of the Crees of Quebec represents the nine Cree communities that comprise the Cree Nation in Quebec, Canada. These Cree bands have since time immemorial lived in the sub-arctic region of the Eastern shore of James Bay. We are indigenous people who hunt, fish and trap as a way of life.

The language of the submission unambiguously demands, with its very first words, international recognition of the land and land-based rights of the eastern James Bay Cree (or *Eeyou'ch,* the Cree term for "people"). Well-being, as I originally found in the ethnographic research that I conducted in one of those nine communities, is similarly an intimate reflection of this assertion of identity as it is defined through historical, familial, cultural, and political connections to the land (Adelson 2000).[1]

The eastern James Bay Cree have been living in, traversing, and sustained by the lands of eastern subarctic Canada for over five thousand years. While the Cree are currently organized into separate communities in northern and north-central Quebec, the relationship to the land that has persisted as hunting, trapping, and fishing remains central to the lives and livelihoods of the Cree people. With the total population now numbering over thirteen thousand in the nine communities, and with Cree maintained as the first language of the eastern James Bay population, the Cree nation is a particularly robust political entity, both provincially and nationally represented by the Grand Council of the Crees (GCC). As I elaborate below, with the signing of a historic treaty in 1975, the Cree became the first self-governing First Nation in Canada and are the beneficiaries of a series of hard-won compensations originally exchanged for over 600,000 km^2 of Cree land.

One of the smallest of the nine Eastern Cree communities is Great Whale, or as it is locally known by its Cree name, Whapmagoostui. Whapmagoostui is a village community located about 1400 kilometers north of the city of Montreal and is a few hundred kilometers beyond the last accessible road in northern Quebec. Situated on a spit of land where the powerful Great Whale River pours into the Hudson Bay, the village site is bordered by these waterways to the south and west, respectively, and, to the immediate north and east by the conifer forests typical of this taiga zone. The waterways and lands that extend many kilometers beyond the village are the traditional hunting grounds of the people of Whapmagoostui. Prior to permanent settlement at this site less than one hundred years ago, the Cree spent most of the year

moving on or across these hunting grounds and trap lines in small familial groups, typically meeting each summer on the south side of the
of the Great Whale River. Although mining activities and, in particular,
the fur trade were already well in existence in Canada in the seventeenth century, neither panned out exceptionally well in this particular region of the country. It was the establishment of a beluga whaling
industry in the river's estuary that firmly established Great Whale as
a post site. The beluga harvested from the river was such a lucrative
resource for the British that it lasted for well over one hundred years.
With the whales hunted to near decimation and with less reliance on
the rendered oil in Great Britain, the whaling industry in this region
came to a halt in the early nineteenth century. The fur trade remained
lucrative enough to have a number of post sites in the region and, by
the mid-1800s, the missionaries began their foray into this sector of the
north. Thus by the time of the cyclical decline in fur-bearing and larger
hunted animals in the first decades of the last century, many of the Cree
(and Inuit) of the surrounding region had already become fairly reliant
on the post and the facilities and services linked to it (Adelson 2000).

The three hundred years after contact was initially made between Cree
and non-Cree, at the height of the Cold War in the 1950s, Great Whale
was selected as one of the early warning radar sites. This seemingly overnight (for the local Eeyou'ch, in particular) transformation of a north-
erly outpost into a fully operational army base firmly secured Whapmagoostui as a settlement location. By the time the base closed down in
1967, many of the Cree people were living and working for extended
periods of time in the village. While the federal government did provide some minimal health and education services to the Native peoples
of Canada as wards of the state, the Cree people were living in dire poverty and without adequate housing or medical services. For the James
Bay Cree, the signing of the James Bay and Northern Quebec Agreement
(JBNQA) in 1975 signaled not only a profound shift in governmental relations with the Cree but also the sustained (if continually hard-fought)
provision of improved health, housing, and educational services.

The JBNQA was the result of a grueling legal battle fought by a small
handful of young Cree leaders and their lawyers against the government
of Quebec and one of its largest corporate industries, Hydro-Quebec.
What began as a government's unilateral announcement of the development of one of the world's largest hydroelectric developments ended
as a social, economic, and political transformation of the Cree people.
With the JBNQA came specific land and financial deals so that Hydro-
Quebec could divert and dam rivers as part of the construction of the
La Grande hydroelectric complex. With the JBNQA also came the legal

basis for the first Native self-government in Canada. Still only a delegated right, the Cree of Quebec now constituted a formal nation with its own governing body. The JBNQA also provides for Cree control of wildlife management, and input into all future environmental impact assessments, as well as administrative control over education, health, local justice, and local and regional governments. As well, the agreement outlines an innovative program of guaranteed income assistance for men and women who live a majority of the year in the bush and who trap and hunt on a full-time basis. Indeed, while everyone—young and old—continues to hunt or participate in bush and camp activities on a regular basis, more than eighty families in Whapmagoostui, for example, still opt to hunt and trap full-time (Masty 2005, 52).[2]

For the people of Whapmagoostui, the JBNQA brought many local changes as a result of this new form of governance and management as well as from the flow of their proportion of the financial settlement into community development and infrastructure. Thus, since the signing of the agreement, this still small community now numbering some eight hundred gained a new band office, clinic, school, new houses (although still not enough for all the families that require them), a hockey arena, new church, new housing for clinic and teaching staff, a youth complex, and a daycare and elder care center. The JBNQA meant, in other words, permanence at this village site that was more clearly than ever before articulated and specifically defined through the legal text of the agreement.

With the announcement of the Great Whale Hydro-Electric Project in 1989, the community of Whapmagoostui and its local and provincial leaders became embroiled for the second time in less than twenty years in a David and Goliath-like struggle against the government of Quebec and Hydro-Quebec. That announcement came just six months into my first arrival in the community to begin a sixteen-month-long ethnographic study of the Cree meaning of "health." Thus, as I have written elsewhere, the looming threat of the project crystallized for many the foundational link between land, well-being, and, by extension, identity (2000). When I interviewed members of the community for that study, they spoke with particular passion about the potential yet unimaginable loss of their land. Already concerned about pollutants and other forms of environmental degradation, the hydroelectric project symbolized an inestimable yet very real and imminent threat to the core of what it meant to be Cree to the members of this community. Being Cree and being well were, I finally came to recognize, as I will elaborate below, one and the same. The project, had it gone forward, would have changed the lives of the people of this still-remote community in immeasurable ways. Fundamentally flawed, the project was—after a long and arduous six-year battle—halted. What did not stop was the way in which the effects of those hydroelectric battles, along with the changing social and political landscape of the Cree nation, influenced the ways in which people articulated the interrelationship between themselves, their land and hunting activities, and their sense of well-being.

Miyupimaatisiiun: The Shifting Landscape of Cree Well-Being

What, for the Cree people, does "well-being" mean? The Cree term *miyupimaatisiiun* best summarizes the elaborate Cree concept of well-being. Because more common English terms such as *being well, living well,* or *health* simply do not capture or reflect the complex particularly of Cree well-being, I purposely translate the Cree term into the more awkward English phrase "being alive well." As much as it might signal the absence of disease, *miyupimaatisiiun* is not just a statement of individual health, nor does it reflect a particular modern morality or economics of health (cf. Foucault 2004). *Miyupimaatisiiun* is the assertion of one's proper sense of place in a broadly defined social and physical Cree landscape. Thus, "being alive well" is the ability to sustain oneself as a member of a Cree community and hence a complex kin and social network. One's social network, in turn, plays a role in the hunt for and distribution of a key food source: bush foods. Bush foods are hunted, trapped, and fished foods, including goose, caribou, beaver, porcupine, rabbit, ptarmigan, duck, fish, and moose. Further, there is a basic and vital connection between the land, its resources, and the Cree people. Bush foods are regularly hunted for primarily by the community's men, and any surplus is distributed to an extended kin network or is saved for future family or community feasts. Thus, for example, when a larger and symbolically more significant animal such as a bear is killed, a special feast will be held with many elders and an extended kin network invited to participate and partake. As well, for most families today, the spring and autumn goose hunts are anticipated as much for the hunt and the goose meat as for the extended period of time spent in the bush. The community of Whapmagoostui will typically empty as most travel out to their respective familial goose hunting camps. With girls and boys learning their respective roles in the hunting process from a young age—including how to maintain a camp and the appropriate respect for the animals' spirits—hunting and bush-related activities remain an important aspect of life for the Cree of Whapmagoostui.[3]

A great deal, however, has changed in the space of a few short decades. While still a very small community, the population has doubled (from four hundred to eight hundred) in just twenty years, with a concomitant burgeoning young population. In terms of hunting and trapping activities, while many families today opt to spend a majority of the year on the land through an income security program, hunting is more typically balanced with the day-to-day life in the village. Employment—whether seasonal, part-time, or regular—raising a family, caring for elderly parents or grandchildren, schooling, and other matters keep most people in the village for the majority of the year. Also, although a majority of the village's older adults were born either in the bush or in Whapmagoostui, today women are regularly flown out of the village to deliver their infants in hospitals away from the community. Young adults now spend more time in the village than on the land or may move away from the village to more urban areas for extended periods to continue their post–high school and advanced studies. Whereas for so many of the older members of the community, the village is defined as one of the places of residence within the larger territorial locations of home, that notion too is changing today. With satellite dishes on so many homes and ready internet access, the community is electronically or digitally connected to the rest of Canada and to the world. Thus, the younger generations live in a village with networks of relations maintained as readily by the internet and air travel as by snowmobile or all-terrain vehicle. Trips onto the land are certainly regular activities, but while hunting and camp life are an intrinsic part of familial and community life, they are experienced as activities distinctly apart from the village.

As much as things have changed locally, a great deal has also transpired at the national level for the Cree, in particular, through the efforts of the Grand Council of the Crees. In 2005, then grand chief Ted Moses announced that "We are now responsible for our future and it is for us to decide what that future will look like" (Moses 2005).[4] This statement was simply inconceivable at the time of either the original La Grande or the Great Whale battles with Hydro-Quebec and the Quebec government. Yet the statement now encapsulates the profound political changes that have taken place in the thirty years since the signing of the JBNQA, and reflects how much has transformed locally, regionally, and internationally for the James Bay Cree.[5] Addressing the Cree 2005 Nation Annual General Assembly, Moses continued:

> We have thrown off the yoke of colonialism through 30 years of struggle and we should now be setting our sights on genuine nation building. Taking up that challenge forces us to address the question of what it is

that defines who we are. We have for a long time been hunters and trappers and we will continue to be hunters and trappers. We will continue to maintain that special relationship with the land. But does being Cree mean being only a hunter and trapper? (2005, 5)

In that seminal address at the end of his term in power, Grand Chief Moses looked back at the past thirty years of nation building as the foundation for a previously unimaginable future for the Cree of northern Quebec. The signing of the 2004 New Relationship Agreement signals a profound change in the relationship between the Cree and Hydro-Quebec.[6] Ending twenty years of legal action between the Cree and Quebec's most significant nationalized industries, the conciliatory new agreement is a move towards a negotiated space for dealings between the Cree nation, the government, and Hydro-Quebec. While this new agreement is certainly not embraced by all, within the context of a host of social health concerns that overwhelm many of the Cree communities and with much concern for the economic prospects for youth, Moses nonetheless sees the Cree nation at the brink of a profound social and political transformation. The Cree are soon to become the majority population in northern Quebec; with the signing of the "Paix des Braves" and New Relationship Agreements with the government of Quebec and Hydro-Quebec, Moses envisions a nation that can participate fully in the economic, political, and social growth of the vast northern region. Are the people of the Cree nation, he asks, ready to relegate the decades upon decades of colonial oppression to history (2005)?[6]

Notions of well-being for the Cree must shift with these shifting concepts of what it means, fundamentally, to be Cree, but will they change as dramatically as Moses is suggesting? Will the concept of *mi-yupimaatisiiun* become a reflection of an idealized past, a marker of a particular historical period that will expire with the passing of this generation of elders? While many do still retain the practices and values inherent in "being alive well", others see such dramatic changes occurring in the younger generations that they can imagine a day when this ideal is lost to an irretrievable past or becomes reified as a relic that one must struggle to preserve. Others, like Ted Moses, view the changes as part of the continuing narrative of the Cree nation. Again, in the words of Moses:

Our way of life has never been a static one, fixed forever in time to be exactly the same thing. There have always been changes—there were many periods before contact with Europeans when we were completely independent, there were adjustments which our ancestors made to accommodate the fur trade, and there were other adjustments when the fur trade began to decrease in importance—and we have continuously adapted ourselves to make beneficial changes for our people. What has endured is our principles and our values. ... Part of the challenge which is facing us now as an indigenous nation is to stay true to the rich and meaningful cultural heritage which we have inherited and to apply it to our current realities and circumstances. The challenge which I believe lies before us is nothing more nor less than a process of reinventing ourselves. This is what our ancestors had to do when faced with new realities and new opportunities and this is now what we need to do (2005, 4).

Drawing on both ageless traditions and contemporary prospects and constraints, Moses is addressing the fundamental tension of a traditionalist perspective. Bush camp, hunting, and related activities reference a particular past and concentrate issues of identity around a specific set of cultural beliefs and practices immediately understood as Cree. If cultural property, activities, and beliefs define the Cree and distinguish them from non-Cree in the face of expansive northern development, there is a risk that "meaningful cultural heritage" will be lost if altered in any way. Thus, if Cree well-being is based on one's relationship to the land and a Cree morality of bush-related activities such that the embodiment of that relationship to the larger social and political processes is epitomized as the ideals of *miyupimaatisiiun*, what becomes of Cree well-being when that relationship changes? Moses suggests that change is not only inevitable but appropriate and to be expected.

Miyupimaatisiiun and Its Changes: In Conversation with a Community Elder

Moving from the national level back to the local, let me reflect on the ways in which the language and practices of Cree well-being are transforming within the community of Whapmagoostui. What follows is an informal question and answer session with a community member with whom I have had a long-standing friendship and professional relationship. The interview is informal in that I did not request community permission to conduct research. Thus it should not be taken as representative of more than one person's perspective and opinion, and offers only a partial glimpse into a complex local reality. These shortcomings notwithstanding, my friend E.M. provides tremendous insight into the present-day situation in Whapmagoostui through personal reflections on some of the trials this community is facing and the concomitant implications for a newly reconfigured sense of *miyupimaatisiiun*.

NA: What has changed in your own life in the last number of years?

EM: I've become a grandparent of four boys. I daresay I've become my mother! I meddle when I get the chance because I have my son, his girlfriend, and their son living with me. This is also one of the changes: the housing situation is still quite bad—people are crowded and the houses can't be built fast enough. In fact, if my other son was in town, I would have both families living with me—and all four young boys—in a three- bedroom house.

NA: What changes stand out the most for you in the community over the last ten years?

EM: In the community, in the last ten years, more teenage pregnancy, more suicides and suicide attempts. There were much fewer attempts not that long ago. There was one who died from sniffing gas. That's what has changed. There are more Inuit and Cree getting together, having babies together. It was quite rare in my time, which has really changed from the old generation. The community is growing, but housing is not and social services also can't cope with the problems. There is a lot of staff turnover in Youth Protection. Since the time you were first here, there has been the addition of a bar that you can go into without being a member—this adds to the problem.

People are also more conscious of "being" Cree; it used to be that they just "lived" but now because of all the other problems creeping in, then they look to their past and say, "this wasn't there in our past—being overweight, alcoholism, diabetes"; and they seem to look for solutions back there, in the past.

There is a swimming pool being built beside the gym—in other words, the facilities are there: the youth center, the hockey arena, the gym, now the swimming pool, and also an elder's facility and a day-care—they are all there, even a new church. These are all changes in the last ten years, but when I think about the youth, there is hardly anyone from the community (some but not enough) doing organized sport or camp activities. Sure, hockey is big—for men and women—but only the school is doing the intramural sports during the school year. No one is doing any summer programs for the youth to do with their culture—bush camp, paddling or portaging expeditions—both cultural and also healthy, and learning the trails and the skills of the people. People would volunteer for this, but there is no money put towards these activities.

I haven't talked much about any good changes. One thing that is good is that there are better health services for people—their health is being monitored closely and the access to specialists in the south is definitely better. Also, it's good that we have all of these facilities, but no one knows how to use them; only hockey is really big and only through school do they have the sports, and usually monitored by teachers. Baseball used to be really big in the summer for both boys and girls, but there is only some organized here and there. Hockey, since we got the arena, has really taken over. But the arena is closed all summer.

In terms of education, the Cree School Board has vocational education in place for those who could not succeed in the regular stream. This is a real improvement in education services. There is a permanent adult education facility in town. There is more access to the adult education program for both adults and youth. But there are still some youth, and their families, who are very traditional and they are being taught the traditional ways most of the year [they are in the bush most of the year and are active trappers]. There was one man working to build a "bush" curriculum for those students going into the bush—in other words, that the bush knowledge would count as vocational education because it would lead to having a livelihood through the Income Security Program—but it was not recognized by the Ministry of Education of Quebec. It's funny that they would recognize a person becoming a janitor, in terms of vocational education, but not a trapper. There are some students who have minor to medium disabilities—they still can become apprentices for the people who live in the bush and get Income Security. The government considers this valid, but they don't recognize the bush education as a vocation.

NA: When I first came to Whapmagoostui, we had long conversations about the stories I was hearing from people and the ways in which people were describing to me their sense of well-being as something very distinctive and very much linked to lives lived on the land. Do you think that this idea of well-being is still prevalent?

EM: As I said, people remember that they were "well" in the past. They remember the peace that they feel out there and being outdoors and moving, that kind of health. And, the ones who now watch TV and speak English, they read about the problems with white man's meat, like mad cow disease and chickens being pumped with steroids, so they look more toward traditional foods when they can. They are more interested in that. The caribou have come back near Great Whale now when they migrate, so people go hunting and get caribou. They don't eat as much store-bought meat/food now, because the caribou are traveling closer to Great Whale and people will go out to hunt them. The women say that they have to do more to cook the caribou meat because the kids enjoy it in stews and other things that take a bit more work to cook [than store-bought foods]! They used to migrate further away, in the old days, the caribou didn't come around their area anymore—that's when people used to speak about the starvation, when the caribou stopped coming around. There is this opportunity now, with the kids who are high school age, they now have a chance to learn how to hunt and how the caribou is butchered and how to clean the skins—it's been happening in the last few years because the caribou are coming around. Even at the cultural camp [a traditional learning center located just to the north of the main village], the younger married men and women are learning to do this—there are programs for them to learn how to tan the caribou skin, and how to make *bimmee* [rendered animal fat] and *pemmican* [a mixture of pulverized dried meat and rendered animal fat] and they have a feast after they are shown how to make the *bimmee*.

NA: Do you think that people now hold this idea of "being alive well" as an ideal or is it something that people strive toward in their daily lives?

EM: People still hold it and strive for it, but when you talk about the young people, they are just being shown these things and whether they are striving for it in their daily lives … I don't think the school children are, except those who are actually in the bush. And, they are there because their parents have chosen to take them out there. The young people, lots of people still go for the spring and fall hunt, so they still seem to like it, but again, because of the changing lifestyles, they need a plane or a 4-wheeler to go. Before families just up and left, and now it's not that accessible to everybody. The younger children don't feel it yet because they are living in town—this is the second generation of kids being raised in town—some of them only go out for the goose hunt. In the past—when you were here, Naomi—the whole town left, it was empty during the goose hunting seasons. Now, about one-third of the town stays back. Maybe it's too expensive to go, maybe there are too many people [to travel to the camp], and for some it's because of health problems that they can't go and someone has to stay with them, and some just can't afford to go.

NA: In what other ways are things changing for the youth today in terms of their idea of well-being? Is it more or less connected to the land and land-based activities? Or, do they have a different sense of well-being?

EM: They are young, they are not raised in the bush, and they live only in the village with all of these facilities, so their life is in Whapmagoostui. They still go in the bush but, using the example of a teenager I know: he goes out to the bush with his family for a few days and then comes back to his house and stays home. I don't know if he is typical, but he is an example of the youth today.

Discussion: Rethinking the Limits of *Miyupimaatisiiun*

E.M.'s discussion of, and especially her sensitivity to the challenges that the youth face today touch upon many interrelated, profound, and at times overwhelming changes that have taken place in her village in the last ten years. While of course providing only a single perspective, E.M. is nonetheless a keen and trusted observer of her community. What she recounts here is disheartening, yet E.M. manages to retain some degree of optimism about the youth, despite troubling conditions unknown in previous generations. What E.M. indicates, too, is that well-being for the youth is not defined so much as by what they are doing, as by how well they can tack between the varying worlds in which they live. For E.M., *miyupimaatisiiun* is, not surprisingly, inextricably tied to bush-related activities and foods, and social networks. The youth, however, are more likely to see the concept of *miyupimaatisiiun* as an ideal; temporally and spatially distant and something they may neither want, nor be able, to attain.

Ted Moses' political speeches, filled as they must be with strategies for success, compellingly articulate the political motivation to move away from an arcane and unrepresentative depiction of Aboriginal peoples as nothing more than traditional. Moses speaks to a future that engages with the far more accurate complex reality of the Cree nation today and with far more optimism than E.M. can muster. Both nonetheless speak to the ways in which the iconic past infuses the present, and to a future that is complexly embedded within the contemporary and ever-changing social, economic, and political landscape of Cree nationhood within the larger nation-state. At both the local and national levels, Cree identity and hence valuation of well-being are viewed as bound to the land and to peoples' sense of their place on it, yet as E.M. tellingly notes: today "people are also more conscious of 'being' Cree; it used to be that they just 'lived' but now because of all the other problems creeping in … they look to their past and say, 'this wasn't there in our past. …'" Indeed, E.M. points to the ways in which Cree well-being is construed less in terms of living on the land than as an abstraction as part of an active engagement in "being Cree" and as against what is understood as being non-Cree (the negative effects of such things as store-bought meat, television, and chronic disease).

Noting that the majority of the youth of today are the second generation to live their lives based in the village itself, E.M. reminds me that the youths' world is profoundly different from the ways in which the community's elders raised their children. Living in the village requires different skill sets and abilities—skills that are not valorized as inherently "Cree." Thus, for those whose lives are increasingly circumscribed by the village borders, there are now specified events and places for the enactment of Cree culture and for an engagement with its language and practices. As the young adults learn, for example, how to skin and tan caribou hides, they are self-consciously engaging in activities that they know are Cree. This practical assertion of being Cree is not new; thirty years of legal battles in which the Cree had to assert their Aboriginal identity and the decades of colonial arrogance that were endured prior to that ensure that many generations of James Bay Cree are able to lay claim to specific beliefs and practices as inherently Cree. What is new, according to E.M., is that the generation of youth who now live in Whapmagoostui must make their own sense of themselves and their ability to "be alive well" as they straddle the increasingly more disparate worlds that exist within the boundaries of their own village. Thus, while not everyone might be able to heed Ted Moses' plea for the Cree to "reinvent" themselves, there is clear recognition at the local level that there is a renegotiation, and hence a shift, in the landscape of Cree well-being. Just as the physical landscape—so vital to previous generations' fundamental conceptualizations of well-being—is a distant locale for the youth of today, the ideals of well-being are transforming into metaphoric landscapes of an increasingly illusory past and a far more complex future.

Much as we must understand that First Nations peoples do not exist in some sort of artificial sphere of either cultural authenticity or decline (cf. Adams 2005), we must similarly recognize that definitions and valuations of concepts such as well-being are neither unitary nor fixed. As important as it is to be recognized as a key and sometimes pragmatic marker of difference, necessary room must always be made to expand, rethink, and alter the meaning of, in this instance, Cree well-being. For the Cree to reinvent themselves, as Moses challenges, is not to inscribe a delimiting concept of identity—nor of well-being—but to engage meaningfully with the all of the nuances and complexities of that world as it transforms, such that both concepts are understood as necessarily always unfinished.

Notes

I am, as ever, indebted to E.M. for our years of conversations and treasure her friendship and her ability to keep me on track. Thank you to Gordon Mathews and Carolina Izquierdo for your thoughtful and valuable editing of earlier versions of this chapter. Any inaccuracies are my own.

1. See Niezen (2000, 2003) for an important discussion of the strategic, political, and symbolic uses of the concept of "indigenous."
2. The Cree traditional lands were significantly reconfigured in 1975 when the James Bay and Northern Quebec Agreement (JBNQA) was signed. After the signing of the 1975 treaty, Cree hunting lands were bounded by parameters spelled out in that agreement. For a complete review of the struggle leading up to the signing of the James Bay Agreement as well as the resultant self-governance agreements, please see Salisbury (1986), Richardson (1977), and the Grand Council of the Cree website (www.gcc.ca).
3. For the Cree, hunting is a negotiation between the animals, their spirits, and the person. Animals will only give themselves up to a hunter and his family if they have acted properly in the bush and in accordance with all of the rules of respect that govern that relationship (Tanner 1979; Adelson 2000). For a fuller discussion of the symbolic and nutritional significance of bush foods and goose hunting, please see Adelson (2000).
4. The grand chief is the head of the Grand Council of the Crees; which is the political body representing all of the James Bay Cree (nine communities). A new grand chief was elected in the fall of 2005.
5. For a discussion of some of the contemporary challenges facing the Cree women, see Adelson n. d.
6. The landmark agreement with Hydro-Quebec emerges out of an earlier and equally historical settlement between the Cree nation and the province of Quebec. The "Paix des Braves" Agreement signals a new conciliatory relationship that builds on the JBNQA; provides a process for settling long-standing disagreements over natural resource management; and is based on cooperative, respectful transactions in all other areas on a nation-to-nation basis. The agreement also paves the way for two new hydroelectric projects in the James Bay Cree territory. The agreement, though, is not without its critics within the Cree communities. Some felt that Moses acted without proper consultation and signed a deal that is not in the people's best interest. Given the years of hostility and impediments to rectifying wrongs that evolved out of the JBNQA, there is good reason to be cautious about this latest deal as well (Gouvernement du Québec 2002; Di Matteo 2002).

References

Adams, Christine. 2005. "Melancholic Attachments: The Making and Medicalisation of Aboriginal 'Loss.'" PhD thesis, Australia National University.

Adelson, Naomi. 2000. *Being Alive Well: Health and the Politics of Cree Well-Being.* Toronto: University of Toronto Press.

————. n.d. Stress Discourse and the Reproduction of Culture: History, Culture, and "Stress" Amongst First Nations Women in a Remote Northern Community. Manuscript.

Bartlett, Judith. 2004. "Conceptions and Dimensions of Health and Well Being for Métis Women in Manitoba," *Circumpolar Health (Nuuk)* 63 (2): 107–13.

Cree Regional Authority, "CRA 2003-4 Annual Report," 2005. http://www.gcc .ca. Accessed 17 April 2006.

Di Matteo, Enzo. 2002. "Damned Deal: Cree Leaders Call Hydro Pact Signed in Secret a Monstrous Sellout." *NOW Magazine Online Edition,* 14 February. http://www.nowtoronto.com/issues/2002-02-14/news_story.php. Accessed 17 April 2006.

Foucault, Michel. 2004. "Crisis of Medicine or Anti-Medicine," trans. E.C. Knowlton, W.J. King, and C. O'Farrell. *Foucault Studies* (ejournal) 1: 5–19. Accessed 12 May 2006

Gouvernement du Québec. 2002. "La 'Paix des Braves' Ouvre la Voie à une Nouvelle Ère de Coopération et de Prospérité Pour la Région de la Baie-James", 7 February. http://www.premier.gouv.qc.ca/general/communiques/ archives_communique/2002/fevrier. Accessed 17 April 2006.

Lock, Margaret and Nancy Scheper-Hughes. 1990. "A Critical-Interpretive Approach in Medical Anthropology: Rituals and Routines of Discipline and Dissent." In *Medical Anthropology: A Handbook of Theory and Method,* ed. T.M. Johnson and C.F. Sargent, 47–72. New York: Greenwood Press.

Mann, Rosemary H. 2005. "Look Wide—Searching for Health in the Borderlands: Experience of Disease Prevention and Health Promotion in a Central Australian Indigenous Settlement." PhD thesis, University of Melbourne.

Masty, David. 2005. "Whapmagoostui," in *CRA Annual Report 2003–4,* 52. http:// www.gcc.ca/pdf/CRA000000001.pdf. Accessed 12 May 2006.

Moses, Ted. 2005. Grand Chief Dr. Ted Moses' Address at the Cree Nation Annual General Assembly in Waswanipi (09/08/05). http://www.gcc.ca Accessed 12 May 2006.

Niezen, Ronald. 2000. "Recognizing Indigenism: Canadian Unity and the International Movement of Indigenous Peoples." *Comparative Studies in Society and History* 42: 119–48.

————. 2003. *The Origins of Indigenism: Human Rights and the Politics of Identity.* Berkeley: University of California Press.

Richardson, Boyce. 1977. *Strangers Devour the Land: The Cree Hunters of the James Bay Area Versus Premier Robert Bourassa and the James Bay Development Corporation.* Toronto: MacMillan.

Salisbury, Richard F. 1986. *A Homeland for the Cree: Regional Developments in James Bay: 1971–1981.* Montreal: McGill-Queen's University Press.

Tanner, Adrian. 1979. *Bringing Home Animals.* St. John's, Canada: ISER Press.

Wilson, Alex. 2004. *Living Well: Aboriginal Women, Cultural Identity and Wellness.* Prairie Women's Health Centre of Excellence Document #79. http://www .pwhce.ca. Accessed 12 May 2006.

PART THREE

WELL-BEING, CULTURE, AND THE STATE

6

WELL-BEING
Lessons from India
Steve Derné

Anthropologists have shown that aspects of the human psyche, like self and emotion, vary because different societies sensitize people to different aspects of human experience. Because of cultural individualism, most middle-class American men feel that they find their "real selves" in pursuing their own individual desires (e.g., Bellah et al. 1985). Because of this focus on the individual, Americans tend to view love as a positive feeling for a special person. In the 1980s, middle-class, upper-caste Indian men living in joint families experienced a more socially oriented cultural milieu: they saw themselves as always entangled in webs of relationships within a group. These Indian men tended to feel that their "real selves" were to be found in following social dictates. These Indian men saw love as a potentially dangerous, individual emotion that might threaten the joint-family structures that supported them.

As Mathews and Izquierdo theorize in this volume, well-being refers to a subjective sense of enduring life satisfaction. Although it is subjective, based on an internal state of mind, well-being is shaped by cultural orientations, as discussed in this volume's introduction and in other chapters. This chapter suggests that because of a sociocentric orientation rooted in a family structure characterized by joint-household living and an economic structure that limits economic independence, the well-being of Indian men such as those I interviewed was rooted in being nourished by group support. For men like these, being forced to support oneself threatened well-being. That these Indian men also felt uneasy without at least some independence suggests that a balance between independence and group guidance is cross-culturally necessary for people to experience well-being. Changes in Indian family and economic structures since the 1980s suggest that it is social structure (rather than a cultural or psychological orientation) that fundamentally grounds standards of well-being, and that social change that transforms culture without a corresponding change in social structure threatens well-being.

Analyzing the Cultural Poles of "Egocentrism" and "Sociocentrism"

Focusing on how the social world is felt and experienced from the subject's point of view, anthropologists have pioneered cross-cultural study of the psyche. Summarizing psychological anthropological research, Shweder (1991, 73) concludes that "cultural traditions and social practices regulate, express, and transform the human psyche, resulting less in psychic unity for humankind than in ethnic divergences in mind, self, and emotion." Since at least Geertz ([1966] 1973, 363), anthropologists have focused on variations in people's self-conceptions. As in many other Western societies, white, middle-class American men's conception of self focuses on the "autonomous individual, presumed able to choose the roles he [or she] will play and the commitments he [or she] will make, not on the basis of higher truths, but according to the criterion of life-effectiveness as the individual judges it" (Bellah et al. 1985, 47). In 1986 and 1987, I interviewed forty-nine upper-caste, middle-class Hindu men, mostly from merchant families ranging in age from their teens to their seventies, who lived and worked in Banaras, India. The interviews, which were conducted in Hindi and lasted from forty minutes to more than two hours, concerned men's ideas about joint-family living, arranged marriages, restrictions on women outside the home, and family interactions within the home. As in many societies that emphasize the sociocentric pole of human social life, these Indians found their "true selves" not in personal, inner experiences but in meeting social and institutional expectations (Derné 1992, 1995).

Anthropologists have a similar tradition of identifying cross-cultural variations in emotions (Lutz 1988; Shweder 1991, 72). Because of their focus on the individual, middle-class Americans tend to regard love as a positive feeling for a unique, special person, and tend to see love as providing individuals with satisfaction and self- development (Swidler 2001). Because they focus on maintaining relationships in a joint family and de-emphasize the individual, the Indian men I interviewed in the 1980s wanted love to follow from duty rather than the specialness of the beloved, and expected that love should be extended toward others in the family, while remaining subordinate to social fear of one's elders (Derné 1995). Thus, when I asked husbands to tell me of their wife's special qualities, they usually insisted she had none. "Whether the wife is good or bad," a married thirty-year-old told me, "she is a member of the family after marriage and for the sake of the relationship, we must certainly love [*mohabbat*] her." These men emphasized that love must not be for an exclusive individual but for "every member of the family."

Phoolchand Mishra, a married twenty-eight-year-old, described Hindi film heroes and heroines as exemplary because their "love [*chahat*] for each other does not minimize their love [*chahat*] for the whole society." By contrast, he said, the Hindi film villain is evil because "he likes the heroine's fleshly beauty alone. He has no concern for the beauty of society." These Indian men commonly described "fear of society" (*samaj ke dar*) as a good moral emotion that prompts correct behavior, and warned that love for one's wife should always be subordinate to such social fear. A newly married man told me that too much love between husband and wife might lead them to consider themselves "great"; such a couple might "become careless and forget their duties toward their families." Love seems to these Hindu men to be a dangerous emotion, threatening to separate the individual from a valued social group.

Lutz (1988) has called attention to variation in "ethnopsychological knowledge systems," cultural variations that play a key part in shaping differences in psyche. All societies have ways of understanding motives that drive action. Despite a diversity of conceptualizations, there are two general types of "frameworks for understanding action" (Derné 1995), one focusing on sources within the individual, the other focusing on sources within the social whole. The self-conceptions and emotions of middle-class American men described above are associated with a society that emphasizes individual motives. As Bellah et al. (1985, 81) put it, many white, middle-class American men are limited by a "language of radical individual autonomy" that sees selves as "arbitrary centers of volition." Because of this, their sense of self is rooted in their individual characteristics, and their notion of love focuses on a feeling for a special, unique individual. The self-conceptions and emotions of Indian men recounted above are associated with a society that scholars widely recognize as de-emphasizing individual volition. Drawing on his clinical work, Kakar (1981, 37) reports that "to size up a situation for oneself and proceed to act upon one's momentary judgment is to take an enormous cultural [and] personal risk. For most Hindus such action is unthinkable." Roland (1988, 252–53) similarly reports that his Indian patients' "central concern" was with "how one's behavior will be regarded by others, particularly by those superior." Most of the men I interviewed in the 1980s focused on the importance of being guided by their social group, especially family elders (Derné 1995). One married twenty-five-year-old eldest son described his reliance on his father by saying that he "wouldn't even do the smallest bit of work without asking father. If the work will be spoiled because he can't be asked, let it get spoiled. We don't do things according to our own mind without asking." At least prior to the advent of globalization, Indian men usually relied on parents to provide guidance about whom to marry and what occupational and educational opportunities to pursue. This socially oriented understanding of human motives supports a sense of self defined by webs of relationships and suggests that love must be a duty-based emotion, extended toward many in a family and subordinated to fear of one's parents.

This paper suggests that such cultural orientations similarly shape standards of well-being. Well-being does not necessarily follow from a fit between personal accomplishments and individual aspirations. In societies such as India, well-being may instead follow from a fit between one's life and significant social expectations.

Middle-class upper-caste Hindu men like those I interviewed in the 1980s can be considered members of a society with shared cultural understandings. I do not intend this term to reference a "whole society" as a conventionally defined political unit, but to instead reference an "instance of prolonged sociation, whatever its boundaries in space or in time" (Collins 1988, 109). To simplify, "culture" refers to the internalized meanings, norms, and values shared within such a society. Men like those I interviewed are in a society that shares a cultural orientation focusing on social obligations rather than individual wants.

But I do not mean to imply that this cultural orientation accurately reflects often individualistic motives, denies individual volition altogether, or is embraced by subordinated groups within broader Indian society. First, sociocentric and egocentric understandings of what drives action should not be confused with actual differences in what influences the actions of individuals. In all societies, both forces external to the individual and forces within the individual have an objective influence on individual actions. What varies cross-culturally is whether one understanding or the other is culturally elaborated (and, thus, whether group control or individual volition is more easily recognized). Individual interests play a part in driving actions of individual Hindu men, even if they see such self-interested actions as directed by the received authority of caste and family. Second, the cultural milieu I focus on may be less common in other regions or among nonmerchants in India, and has never been fully shared by lower-caste Indians (Khare 1984) or Indian women (Derné 2000, 339–43). Because of their placement in the social structure, these groups have long tended to have a more individualistic orientation. Third, the sociocentric orientation of men like those I interviewed has also long been balanced by "second languages," which, while less rich and familiar, have allowed even men like those I interviewed to understand their own individual desires. Nor should we assume that a sociocentric cultural orientation has persisted in the face of globalization since the 1980s, which has changed the structural realities faced by men like those I interviewed. Rather, the cultural understandings I describe are characteristic of particular social arrangements of a particular time and place.

Group Guidance as a Basis of Well-Being

In chapter 7, Jankowiak shows that communist authoritarian social organization undermines people's well-being by stunting their control over their environment. But one should not assume that all members of the human species have a physical need to feel in control of their situation. Rather, in a sociocentric social milieu, humans experience well-being when guided by others and may feel a loss of well-being when forced to rely on their individual selves to control a situation.

The men I interviewed in the 1980s tended to view legitimate action as guided by an individual's social group (Derné 1995). They repeatedly referred to honor and tradition to justify family practices like arranged marriages, joint-family living, and relations between family members. By declaring that they act honorably or that tradition is motivating their actions, these men described their actions as appropriate for any member of their social group, rather than being motivated by individual inclination. A married thirty-two-year-old Brahman justified arranged marriages by saying, "we have to move under whatever is the family's society. … Whatever customs are there in the society of Brahmans, we move according to those customs." These men often felt that established customs must be followed, whatever they may be. A married thirty-five-year-old who commented that women go outside more now than they did in his youth refused to consider which arrangement was right, saying that "whatever situation is moving right now is right." These men prefer to be guided by their elders. One man I interviewed, Phoolchand Mishra, says that "father's opinions are given the main importance. Our mental state is that all problems are solved in the way father says."

These men experienced well-being in being guided and nourished by others, more than in being in control of a situation. Men often referred to the pleasures of being supported by parents. In describing why he married according to his parents' wishes, Phoolchand Mishra said, "Now, you are seeing what kind of friendship I have with my father. The relationship is good because I married according to my parents' liking. If I had gone according to my own mind, father would feel hurt and would not take any interest in solving my problems." Phoolchand experiences well-being because his family is there to assist him: "When the marriage happens by the liking of the parents, a big form of society is always ready to cooperate in every way." Tej Gupta, twenty-one, is an eldest son who lives with his parents, brothers, and sisters, and three uncles and their families; he is a college graduate who expects to be married soon. When I mentioned the possibility of living separate from his parents, Tej recoiled and exclaimed that "the biggest difficulty of living separately is that one has left one's parents." For Tej, it is a "great pleasure" [*anand*] to live in a family with his parents: "In our home, food is cooked and eaten together. If anyone has any trouble, they bear it together." Vinod Gupta, a thirty-four-year-old living in a family with his parents, wife, and brothers' families, similarly describes the joint family as providing "a very happy life. As much love [*pyar*] as one gets in the joint family one could never get living alone." For Vinod, like many other men, joint-family living is a source of security: "What security one gets in the joint family one will not get living separately. The feeling of insecurity is very much among those that live separately."

This focus on being guided by others extends outside family to business relations (Kakar 1981, 119; Sinha 1990). Roland (1988, 36) found, for instance, that his Indian patients relied on "active support, respect and involvement of senior authority figures" at work and felt uneasy without such support.

Because of the desire to be nurtured by others, some men experienced a lack of well-being when cut off from such nurturance. Anil Gupta, seventy-six, operates a tobacco shop and lives with one of his sons, near his other sons. Anil is an only child whose mother died when he was an infant, leaving him with just his father and grandmother. Anil felt intensely uneasy when his father and grandmother died:

> I became completely helpless. Even for an ordinary thing, I had to act according to my own mind! Because I didn't have any relatives, there was no one to advise me. I did whatever came into my mind with whatever results! The situation was very terrible because when I looked around my neighborhood I saw that someone had two brothers, someone else had three brothers and some others had four brothers. Then, this came into my heart: 'How unfortunate I am because I don't have anyone!'

Psychoanalysts Kakar (1981, 20–21) and Roland (1988, 103) report that unease at being separated from their joint family is common among male Indian patients. Rather than providing a sense of well-being, being forced to act on one's own is profoundly disturbing.

The uncertainty men felt when contemplating living separately highlights that well-being depends on having someone to guide them. Phoolchand Mishra commented that the family of a boy who marries for love "becomes indifferent" to the boy and "sees him with a hateful look."

Because of this "anger," they "separate" the son, "abandoning him to himself." The disgust Phoolchand showed in describing this possibility suggests that such abandonment is a horribly frightening possibility. Ashok Mishra, a married twenty-six-year-old, can barely imagine the "difficulties" he would face living separately from his parents: "If a person lives alone, he will either do bad things or he will commit suicide." Prem Singh, a twenty-four-year-old eagerly awaiting his marriage, recognized the difficulty of "controlling" himself when it comes to "matters of sex." By living with his parents, he says, he has the "emotional calculation that my parents are above me. There is somebody to guide me and I am under somebody." Prem imagines that college students are instead "hunted" by their own bad thoughts that they are "free." For men like Prem and Ashok, being situated where they can be guided by others seems a key basis of well-being.

Indeed, men seem to experience a loss of well-being when their own desires move them to act against social pressures. Many men handled this by altering their actions to conform with social demands. Krishna Das Singh, twenty-five, described himself as "hating" the woman his parents wanted him to marry. Krishna broke "all the pots and pans in the house and reject[ed] the marriage hundreds of thousands of times." But ultimately Krishna felt compelled to marry due to his parents' appeals to family honor:

> I was compelled to marry although I had no liking for the girl then and I do not like her to this day. My parents started to say "our honor will go. We have fixed the marriage." … I [began to] think that if I left her, there would never be any honor for her in society. … I thought that I should not cause problems. I thought, "let's go anyway. I will manage."

Krishna is disturbed that his failure to follow expectations would harm his wife and cause his family dishonor. Having finally accepted his wife, Krishna described himself as happy that he now fulfils his role as husband, although he still dislikes his wife:

> Whatever I have got I have passed with her and have fulfilled my roles according to my capacity. I don't act as if I don't like my wife. I do everything for her when it comes to food, drink and clothing. … Everybody thinks that I like my wife but I don't like her.

Krishna was disturbed when his actions conflicted with pressure from his parents. Having bowed to their wishes, Krishna finds well-being, focusing on the security he gets in a joint family:

> Today, my brother may have food and money when I have none. We can both live from what he earns. If my brother does not have these things,

then I can feed him. ... If I am ill and cannot walk around, brother can look after me and show me to the doctor. When I become well again, I can show him to the doctor.

Nandu Gupta, thirty-five, was similarly distressed at the marriage his parents arranged for him. For the first eighteen months of marriage, he refused any relationship with his wife. Nandu was so upset that his wife's father was "approaching everyone saying, 'you have to make him understand that ... he should not leave her.'" One day, Nandu threw a plate in his wife's face, injuring her. But Nandu's wife denied having been beaten, a devotion that gave Nandu "inspiration." "What fault has she done?" he asked himself. When he saw an educated man with a handicapped wife at a temple, he had a "feeling" [*bhavna*] that his own wife was better than that. "After that," Nandu says, his "love [*prem*] for her became very deep." Like Krishna, Nandu was distressed when his own happiness conflicted with social demands, harming others who were following social expectations. Like Krishna, Nandu gained a sense of well-being by bowing to those demands.

Having emphasized group guidance, however, we must not deny the complementary pleasures of being an individual. Experiencing one's own wants is as universal an experience as being nurtured by social groups (Heelas 1981). When societies emphasize social duty, people are prompted to become aware of the opposite pole of experience—those who break free from social duty (Hewitt 1989, 72). Among the men I interviewed in the 1980s, a "first language" (Bellah et al. 1985) of being guided by social groups is complemented by a "second language" that recognizes people's individual desires. While less rich, familiar, and legitimate, this second language nonetheless helped many men recognize their own wants (Derné 1995). Most of these men focus most on the pleasures of living in larger groups, but many also recognize that for well-being, larger groups must not crush their own pursuits.

Many men emphasized how group guidance must be tempered by recognition of individual family members' autonomy. Rajendra Gupta, a twenty-eight-year-old living with his wife, parents, and younger brother's family, values living in a joint family, but also a degree of independence:

It's not right if everything is dependent on the parents. It's wrong if you have to ask for five rupees. The joint family is right if you can spend your money and roam around as you like. The joint family is wrong if there is force from the parents for everything—that one should not go to the movies, or should not go moving around.

Deepak Mishra, thirty, similarly focuses on the importance of freedom within the family. While emphasizing that his father is the *malik* [head],

Deepak says that "since the family is full of adults, the *malik* does not obstruct us in any way. We are free to do whatever we want—roam around, see films, whatever." An emphasis on compromise is a common way that men balance their desire to make their own choices with their desire to be safely guided by their families. Sunil Gupta, a thirty-five-year-old living in a family headed by his elder brother, accepts that he and his brothers should always "tell our thoughts to the *malik* and listen to his talk." But he emphasizes that "somewhere he is flexible and somewhere we are flexible." While the primary source of well-being was nourishment by a larger family, most men also needed opportunities to follow their individual desires as well.

Structure, Culture, and Psyche

I have discussed how a sociocentric cultural milieu largely shapes well-being, but what are the sources of this milieu? Much of my previous work has aimed to show that social structure—how society is organized—shapes cultural and psychological orientations (Derné, 1995, 2000, 2005a). As Swidler (2001, 176) puts it, cultural "consistencies across individuals come less from common inculcation by cultural authorities than from the common dilemmas institutional life poses in a given society. Not shared indoctrination, but shared life-structuring institutions create the basis of a common culture." Thus, the individualistic cultural orientation of many middle-class American men makes sense given an economic structure that provides opportunities and autonomy and a family structure that offers individuals choice about marriage. The more sociocentric orientation of the Indian men I interviewed in the 1980s made sense given economic structures that gave young men few opportunities for independence, pushing them to rely on parental support. These men's focus on love as duty-based made sense given the institutional reality of arranged marriages, while their focus on love as tempered by social fear made sense given a social structure in which young couples lived in joint families and relied on these families for economic support (Derné 1995, 2000). Needing the joint family to provide economic security, men emphasized the goodness of love that reflects in many directions because this focus helped bind members of a joint family together. Men emphasized the importance of being guided by social fear because this orientation tempered the intense passions between husband and wife that might fracture the joint family. While Shweder (1991, 73) is right to recognize how "psyche and culture ... live together, require each other, and dynamically, dialectically and jointly make each other up," social structure ultimately grounds cultural meanings and psychological orientations.

A sense of well-being for the men whom I interviewed in the 1980s was grounded in group support partly because of a broad-based cultural orientation. Focusing on how the "Hindu world image" has "decisively influenced" Indian ways of thinking, Kakar (1981, 15–37) emphasizes how Hinduism urges individuals to stay true to the "particular life task" defined by their dharma. The Indians Shweder (1991, 220) interviewed regarded dharma as "an independently existing and objective reality, somewhat like the law of physics" — and Shweder notes that to understand this law, the people he interviewed often turned to respected authorities. Kakar (1981, 21) argues that cultural emphasis on *moksha* (release) focuses on undoing the distinction between self and other. A deeply rooted, widespread cultural orientation may, then, shape Indians to find well-being in following social guidance while de-emphasizing individual striving.

But shared experiences in life-structuring institutions, like family and economy, are probably more important in making group guidance fundamental to these men's notion of well-being. Eighty percent of the men I interviewed lived in families with more than one married couple; about half lived in families with three or more married couples. While this may be more common than in India as a whole, many Indian couples spend the early years of married life in households headed by their parents or brothers. The joint-family institution gives people a sense that they can rely on others for support. Because in a joint family, a mother's care is complemented by other caretakers (siblings, aunts, uncles, grandparents), infants' needs are consistently met and dependency is prolonged (Derné 2000; Seymour 1993). Because of this prolonged mode of mothering in which an infant's every demand is met, Kakar (1981, 104), Roland (1988, 232–33), and Seymour all conclude that Indian men have only weakly differentiated selves and see themselves as deeply connected to others. As Seymour (1993, 59) concludes, "prolonging a child's physical dependence on others" creates a "sense of interdependence in a society that does not value independence." The institutional structure of joint families that provides multiple caretakers creates a preference to rely on others, but ongoing interactions in a joint-family reinforce this preference. A forty-four-year-old described how

> when any tensions arise [in the family], we sit together, think, and solve the problem. ... If my younger brother did something wrong, then all four brothers say to him, "You are doing wrong." This has a mental effect on him [and] ... he comes again to his place.

Interactions such as these are made possible by joint-family living and reinforce the notion that one can rely on one's family.

Men's focus on family support as critical to their well-being also follows from the economic structures within which they live. Perhaps because most of the men I interviewed in the 1980s played roles in family businesses, they often talked of the material difficulties of trying to live without familial support. But in the 1980s, even nonmerchants usually married before they were economically self-supporting and relied on parents in the early years of married life. The men I interviewed talked of how joint-family living provided honor and practical support—issues important for nonmerchants as well. As Kakar (1981, 121) emphasizes, lack of government programs of unemployment compensation and old-age benefits makes family key to social security. Economic structures that limit young wage earners' independence and that fail to provide a safety net pushed people to rely on their families, a structural reality that shapes standards of well-being.

Bourdieu identifies social structures as having a double existence: structures exist not just in the material world of institutions, but are internalized in the "conduct, thought, feelings, and judgments" of social agents (Bourdieu 1992, 7–18). While Bourdieu's (1992, 12–13) terminology differs from mine, he highlights the fact that exposure to particular social structures instills dispositions in individuals that internalize the necessities of the social environment. Joint-family structures that institutionalize family support and economic structures that provide only tenuous financial independence push toward a cultural and psychological need for family support.

It is worth noting here that the orientation of Indian women may differ from that of men because of their different situation within the structural realities of family life. While men focus on maintaining joint-family harmony, Raheja and Gold (1994, 20) emphasize that women's oral culture recognizes "the desirability of disrupting patrilineal unity in favor of a focus on conjugality." Moore (1995, 290) shows that while men tend to rely on family authority, women's moral reasoning focuses more on personal interests. Puri (1998, 442) shows that women who read romances value "independent thinking" and "self reliance." Women may develop this greater sense of independence because they do not live within one family through their lives, but move to their husband's family on marriage. As Lamb (1997, 289–90) puts it, "women's personhood is unique in that their ties are disjoined and then remade, while men's ties are extended and enduring." Because a husband is her best ally in a family in which she is expected to do most of the work, a young wife focuses on cultivating an exclusive one-on-one relationship with her husband so that he might intervene to improve her life (Derné 2000, 342–43). Given their different location within the joint-family institution, young wives may find well-being not in maintaining a broader family, but rather in separating from it. Focusing on these Indian women highlights how much external structural realities influence people's internal senses of and strategies for well-being.

Social Change and Well-Being

A fit tends to develop between social structures and the cultural and psychological orientations (including a sense of well-being) that support them. In the 1980s, joint-family structures and economic structures that limited individuals' opportunity for economic security supported a cultural and psychological orientation emphasizing well-being as found in family support. People within this orientation tended to act in ways that reproduced the existing structures of economy and family. Because they found well-being in being guided by others, they wanted to live in joint families and did not press to increase individual opportunities in the economy. In stable times, people tend to experience well-being because a fit develops between their cultural and psychological orientation and the social structures with which they live.

Transformations in cultural understandings and/or structural patterns may disrupt this fit, threatening well-being. In the years since I conducted the interviews I focus on above, the Indian economy has opened, increasing opportunities for those with skills that are marketable in the global economy. New media have become widely available, expanding the family possibilities that Indians can imagine. How might these changes be transforming well-being?

Until the mid-1980s, India pursued autonomous economic development with limited global entanglements. When the oil price rise associated with the 1991 Gulf War led to a foreign-exchange crisis, the Indian government turned to the IMF, which demanded reduced restrictions on investment, devaluation of the rupee, and the lifting of foreign-exchange controls. Within five years, imports more than doubled (Shurmer-Smith 2000, 21–25). The transnational movement of media followed economic liberalization, as cable television offerings suddenly competed with state-run television and Hollywood films competed with local Hindi films. The number of television channels grew from one state-run channel in 1991 to more than seventy cable channels in 1999. Access to television increased from less than 10 percent of the urban population in 1990 to nearly 75 percent by 1999. In 1991, cable television reached

300,000 homes; in 1999, it reached 24 million homes. India remains the world's largest producer of feature films, but with the easing of foreign-exchange restrictions, Hollywood captured 10 percent of the market (Thussu 2000).

Newly introduced cultural ideals, by disrupting the fit between structural realities and existing cultural ideals, may threaten well-being. New media might create new desires for consumption that cannot be met through existing economic structures, or new desires for love that cannot be met through family arrangements based on arranged marriages and joint-family living. Liechty (2002, 39) describes how Ramesh, a Nepali youth, became "aware of limitations of his life as a Nepali" because "foreign media … constantly … bring up images of 'America,'" which Ramesh compared to the "extreme deprivation" that he saw in his own life. Liechty (2001, 43–46) describes how the growth of foreign pornography in Nepal led men to develop new desires, which threatened the well-being of their wives. Because of these films, one woman complained, "in what a bad manner [men] think of others! Even their own sisters they begin to look at in this way!" Another said that because of the films, "men want sex all the time. … They think that if we watch it, it will affect us, [but] … women aren't so interested in this." In Nepal, which has also experienced an opening economy accompanied by new media, new cultural images have created desires that threaten the well-being of those whose lifestyles are inconsistent with these images.

While new media may threaten well-being by creating new desires that economic possibilities can never fulfill, my research suggests that men like those I interviewed tend to reject media messages that are beyond their structural possibilities. In 2001, I interviewed thirty-two male filmgoers in Dehra Dun, India, replicating a study that I had conducted in India in 1991 (Derné 2005a, 2005b). The men I interviewed ranged in age from their teens to their thirties; they were students, professionals, self employed, or holders of lower-middle-class jobs. Because they lacked English-language skills and global connections, new high-paying jobs linked to new global markets were out of reach. Yet, cultural globalization dramatically changed the media landscape these men encountered. In 1991, no Hollywood film screened in the three months I worked in Dehra Dun; in 2001, dubbed Hollywood films were the main fare at the city's two elite theatres. While in 1991, none of the men I asked had seen Hollywood films, in 2001, nearly 60 percent had. In 1991, cable television was unavailable, but a decade after economic liberalization, almost 70 percent of those I interviewed had access to cable television.

Yet despite the transformed media landscape and the increased celebration of cosmopolitan lifestyles, the men I interviewed in 2001 remain as committed to arranged marriages as the men I interviewed before the global media deluge. New media did not create new, unfulfilled desires that threaten well-being. Instead, given structural realities, men simply rejected the messages they saw on the screen as fantasies. Vinod, an unmarried twenty-two-year-old, enjoys cable television and Hindi film love stories, but remains committed to arranged marriage: "Love marriages are only stories in films. In real life they are not possible. I haven't given a thought to marriage, but I know I'll marry according to my parents' wishes."

This mantra was voiced by the range of ordinary middle-class men I interviewed. Virendra, twenty-two, a postgraduate engineering student living with his parents, likes to copy the "smart dress" of his favorite heroes and enjoys Hindi film love stories, but he too remains committed to arranged marriage: "In reality, [love marriages] are not successful. In actual life, a love marriage is not possible. I'll marry with my parents' wishes." Another nineteen-year-old student living in a joint family headed by a father with a good service job similarly said that while the films he likes are "love stories, that wouldn't be possible in real life. … Any girl I could find for myself would not be as good as the girl my parents will find for me." Despite a decade of imported mass media celebrating the search for love, similar percentages of men in my two surveys voiced disapproval of love marriages (15 of 22 in 1991 and 21 of 32 in 2001). A 1998–1999 study found that 65 percent of fifteen to thirty-four-year-olds in Delhi, Mumbai, Kanpur, and Lucknow said that they would obey their elders "even if it hurts" (Page and Crawley 2001, 176). Abraham's (2001, 49–151) 1996–1998 study found that a majority of low-income students in Mumbai "preferred an arranged marriage for its stability and security." Despite the new media messages of independence, well-being remains rooted in family and economic structures that institutionalize group guidance.

Television and films today celebrate consumerism and Western brand names (Derné 2005a). Because these new messages have been accompanied by the new availability of goods, the filmgoers I interviewed in 2001 find in consumerism a new source of well-being. One self-employed man is proud to own a motorcycle and hopes to be able to buy an automobile within five years. Many men are happy with consumer items like televisions and cosmopolitan fashion: they enjoy showing off jeans and brand-name logos as they promenade around cinema halls. A prosperous, unmarried thirty-year-old who lives with his parents and brothers and their families says he sees films "for a bit of fashion." This focus on consumerism trickles far down the class hierarchy. Osella and Osella (2000, 119–20) show that even poor, lower-caste men participate in the consumer world by sporting baggy pants and shirts with extravagant designs. Shop owners in Banaras report great demand in T-shirts and jeans due to TV advertisements and serials (Page and Crawley 2001, 160). New celebrations of consumerism don't threaten well-being because economic structures increased the availability of consumer goods, allowing people to satisfy new desires.

But some are uneasy about the new images, for reasons similar to the Nepali women who are threatened by pornography. Some men I interviewed feared new media would threaten the family arrangements they prefer. Virendra, twenty-two, wants an arranged marriage and enjoys living in a joint family headed by his police-officer father and full-time mother. He likes cosmopolitan styles, but is uneasy about the influence of cosmopolitan media. He complains that India has changed because satellite television "is making the younger people too mature. During my earlier years, I didn't know what kids know today." Umesh, a civil draftsman whose marriage has just been arranged, believes that Hindi films should teach "how a sister and brother should relate or how an ideal son should relate to his parents." While Umesh likes Hollywood films and enjoys satellite television in the household he shares with his parents, he is disturbed that new programming gives the message that "a brother should allow his sister to go with her boyfriend to watch a movie. These are not good things," he says, "so they shouldn't be shown on television." Mankekar (2004, 417) similarly reports that the lower-middle-class men and women she interviewed were excited by satellite television, but also felt "anxiety" that new media would "erode … Indian culture." Such concerns about how global media images might disrupt local gender arrangements have been the source of protests against new media. In protesting Valentine's Day, activists in Delhi and Kanpur attacked couples in restaurants and forced them to flee. Protesters targeted the 1996 Indian staging of the Miss World pageant as a threat to Indian womanhood because of its embrace of immodest fashion (Oza 2001, 1067). Protesters have sometimes succeeded in stopping cable serials that they find offensive (Oza 2001, 1072). The uneasiness about new gender imaginations that drive these protests suggests that new media may not threaten well-being by creating new desires that can't be fulfilled, but instead by challenging people's conviction that arrangements they prefer will be able to endure.

Threats to well-being, then, seem to occur when social change disrupts the fit between cultural understandings and structural arrangements. Some people, like the youth Liechty describes, embrace new cultural media and experience a loss of well-being when they can't fulfill new desires. But for the men I interviewed, new cultural celebrations of consumerism do not threaten well-being because changing structural arrangements allow them to consume more global products. New cultural celebrations of love and independence tend to be rejected because continuing economic and family structures strongly support existing cultural notions that focus on group guidance. But like the Nepali women Liechty describes, the male filmgoers I interviewed experience threatened well-being because of their uneasiness that others might reject lifestyles that they feel committed to because of their cultural understandings, psychological dispositions, and the structural realities that they face.

Implications for Understanding Well-Being

What are the implications of this analysis for understanding well-being? First, like self and emotion, the basis of well-being is culturally constructed and varies from place to place. The men I interviewed in the 1980s found well-being more in being guided by nurturing groups than in taking initiative to pursue individual goals.

Second, Indian men's grounding of well-being in group guidance highlights that a felt sense of well-being depends on the well-being of others. Well-being arises when one's life matches one's wants, but to speak of "achievements" and "personal aspirations" makes one's wants far too individualistic and self-centered, neglecting that "achievements" that harm others may threaten one's own well-being. Thus, Nandu Gupta and Krishna Das Singh, who initially opposed marriages their parents arranged for them, could not experience well-being as long as their actions were harming their families' honor or injuring blameless women whom they were to marry.

For many indigenous people, well-being can only occur so long as each individual's life doesn't harm other individuals or natural processes on which life depends. The Hawaiian elders interviewed by Holmes (forthcoming) recognize that money is peripheral to real abundance, which comes from the ability to live from the land. One elder told of a Hawaiian who refused offers of money to dam the water's land because the water ultimately provided life. The Hawaiian activists who protested the US Navy's bombing of the island of Kaho'olawe could feel no well-being so long as the land was being injured—the land they see as the source of life.

Religious conceptions originating in India recognize that well-being only comes with health of both self and environment. Buddhism's focus on the interconnections of all things suggests that one can only experience well-being if one's actions do not harm others. Indians' worship of trees and plants reflects a cosmology that holds person and nature are inseparable (Shiva 1989, 40). Thus, Indians participating in the Chipko movement could not experience well-being as long as there was a threat to life-giving trees. Seeing forests as bearing "soil, water, and pure air," Chipko women's well-being was threatened by the destruction of forests that they regarded as essential to maintaining life in India. That social movements to overcome caste oppression so often focus on improving the status of the group (by, for instance, converting to Buddhism) (e.g., Juergensmeyer 1982) suggests dissatisfaction flows as much from the perception that one's group is threatened as from individual difficulties. Indeed, to some extent in all societies, the subjective sense of well-being may extend beyond an assessment of one's individual life, focusing as well on other people or on the natural environment with which one is interconnected.

Third, the basis of well-being tends to be rooted in structural arrangements and cultural understandings. The men whom I interviewed found well-being in group guidance because of a cultural focus on how selves are embedded in webs of relationships, a cultural focus that itself rested on structural arrangements like joint-family living, arranged marriages, and an economy that could not provide security to individuals. Indians found well-being in support from family because the economy could provide only tenuous security, while joint-family living was a common arrangement that supported individuals. Living with these social arrangements, Indian men found well-being in situations in which others provided for their needs.

Fourth, well-being is threatened when social changes disrupt the fit between cultural understandings, structural arrangements, and psychological wants that are the basis of well-being. For the filmgoers I interviewed in 2001, new cultural ideas challenged well-being by appearing to threaten preferred stable lifestyles. But well-being does not face much threat when cultural changes, like the celebration of consumerism, are coupled with structural changes, such as the flourishing open economy, that allowed people to act on new desires. It is correct to suggest that well-being arises from a fit between a person's aspirations and a person's accomplishments; but we must recognize that aspirations are shaped by macro-level cultural ideas, while the possibility of achievement is shaped by macro-level social structures. Because a fit often develops between cultural ideals and structural possibilities, feelings of well-being are common. But when social change transforms cultural understandings without transforming structural realities or transforms structures without a simultaneous transformation in cultural priorities, dissatisfaction is likely.

Fifth, while I have focused on the social construction of well-being, balance between individual achievements and group support appears cross-culturally necessary for well-being. Being supported and nourished by their families was the fundamental basis of well-being for the men I interviewed in the 1980s. But for such social support to be truly satisfying, men also needed opportunities to fulfill their own individual desires. American society celebrates individual achievement, so individual striving is a fundamental basis of many middle-class Americans' well-being. Yet Putnam's research (2000, 385) shows that "depth of one's social connections" is associated with Americans' life satisfaction, suggesting that ties to others are a necessary complement to individual pursuit of goals.

Unduly influenced by individualistic cultural assumptions of consumer capitalist societies, scholars of well-being are wrong to identify an individual's control of a situation as fundamental to well-being. A focus on the middle of the life course also reflects a bias in these studies. Vatuk (1990, 68) shows that the elderly in India "professed general satisfaction" and "well-being" when they are cared for and served by other family members. She reports that while "American elderly people unable to conform to our cultural ideal of self reliance" sometimes felt "shame or guilt," Indian elders typically felt content that their offspring supported them "in comfort with grace and loving concern." Studies of well-being that assume the universal importance of individual control and autonomy reflect the assumptions of the earning years of a consumerist capitalist society.

Focusing on more socially oriented societies such as India shows that scholars should not assume that well-being flows mostly from individual achievements. Given cultural assumptions and structural realities, many people instead find well-being in the support of others. It appears, moreover, that the pleasures of reliance on social support may be a human universal that anthropologists should consider as a component of well-being in even the most individualistic of societies.

Notes

I am grateful to Gordon Mathews for inviting and commenting on this essay. I am especially grateful for the comments of William Jankowiak. I have been unable to address all of his concerns and I am sure he would disagree with many of my conclusions, but his comments helped me strengthen the argument and suggested important directions for my future work. Because this essay draws on studies conducted over fifteen years, it is difficult to single out all of the institutions that have supported the research, but the most important ones include the American Institute of Indian Studies, the US Department of Education, the Rockefeller Foundation, SUNY–Geneseo, and Delhi University. The research depended on many research assistants, the most important of whom include Narendra Sethi, Nagendra Gandhi, Parvez Khan, and A. Ramchandra Pandit.

References

Abraham, Leena. 2001. "Redrawing the *Lakshman Rekha*: Gender Differences and Cultural Constructions in Youth Sexuality in Urban India." *South Asia* xxiv: 133–56.
Bellah, Robert N., Richard Madsen, William M. Sullivan, Ann Swidler, and Steven M. Tipton. 1985. *Habits of the Heart: Individualism and Commitment in American Life*. New York: Harper and Row.
Bourdieu, Pierre. 1992. *An Invitation to Reflexive Sociology*. Chicago: University of Chicago Press.
Collins, Randall. 1988. "The Durkheimian Tradition in Conflict Sociology." In *Durkheimian Sociology*, ed. Jeffrey Alexander, 107–28. Cambridge: Cambridge University Press.
Derné, Steve. 1992. "Beyond Institutional and Impulsive Conceptions of Self: Family Structure and the Socially Anchored Real Self." *Ethos* 20: 259–88.
———. 1995. *Culture in Action: Family Life, Emotion, and Male Dominance in Banaras, India*. Albany: SUNY Press.
———. 2000. "Culture, Family Structure and Psyche in Hindu India: The 'Fit' and the 'Inconsistencies.'" *International Journal of Group Tensions* 29, no. 3/4: 323–48.
———. 2005a. "The (Limited) Effect of Cultural Globalization in India: Implications for Culture Theory." *Poetics* 33: 33–47.
———. 2005b. "Globalization and the Making of a Transnational Middle Class: Implications for Class Analysis." In *Critical Globalization Studies*, ed. William I. Robinson and Richard Appelbaum, 177–86. New York: Routledge.
Geertz, Clifford. [1966] 1973. "Person, Time and Conduct in Bali." In *The Interpretation of Cultures*. New York: Basic, 360–411.
Heelas, Paul. 1981. "The Model Applied: Anthropology and Indigenous Psychologies." In *Indigenous Psychologies: The Anthropology of the Self*, ed. Paul Heelas and Andrew Lock, 39–64. New York: Academic Press.
Hewitt, John. 1989. *Dilemmas of the American Self*. Philadelphia: Temple University Press.
Holmes, Leilani. Forthcoming. *Ancestry of Experience: A Journey into Hawaiian Ways of Knowing*. Honolulu: University of Hawaii Press.
Juergensmeyer, Mark. 1982. *Religion as Social Vision: The Movement Against Untouchability in 20ᵗʰ Century Punjab*. Berkeley: University of California Press.
Kakar, Sudhir. 1981. *The Inner World: A Psycho-analytic Study of Childhood and Society in India*. 2nd ed. Delhi: Oxford University Press.
Khare, Ravindra S. 1984. *The Untouchable as Himself: Ideology, Identity and Pragmatism among the Lucknow Chamars*. New York: Cambridge University Press.

Lamb, Sarah. 1997. "The Making and Unmaking of Persons: Notes on Aging and Gender in North India." *Ethos* 25: 279–302.

Liechty, Mark. 2001. "Women and Pornography in Kathmandu: Negotiating the 'Modern Woman' in a New Consumer Society." In *Images of the 'Modern' Woman in Asia: Global Media, Local Meanings*, ed. Shoma Munshi, 34–54. Richmond, UK: Curzon.

———. 2002. "'Out Here in Kathmandu': Youth and the Contradictions of Modernity in Urban Nepal." In *Everyday Life in South Asia*, ed. Diane P. Mines and Sarah Lamb, 37–47. Bloomington: Indiana University Press.

Lutz, Catherine A. 1988. *Unnatural Emotions: Everyday Sentiments on a Micronesian Atoll and Their Challenge to Western Theory*. Chicago: University of Chicago Press.

Mankekar, Purnima. 2004. "Dangerous Desires: Television and Erotics in Late Twentieth Century India." *Journal of Asian Studies* 63: 403–31.

Moore, Erin. 1995. "Moral Reasoning: An Indian Case Study." *Ethos* 23: 286–327.

Osella, Filippo and Caroline Osella. 2000. *Social Mobility in Kerala: Modernity and Identity in Conflict*. London: Pluto.

Oza, Rupal. 2001. "Showcasing India: Gender, Geography, and Globalization." *Signs* 26: 1067–95.

Page, David and William Crawley. 2001. *Satellites Over South Asia*. New Delhi: Sage.

Puri, Jyoti. 1997. "Reading Romance Novels in Postcolonial India." *Gender & Society* 11: 434–52.

Putnam, Robert D. 2000. *Bowling Alone: The Collapse and Revival of American Community*. New York: Simon and Schuster.

Raheja, Gloria Goodwin and Ann Grodzins Gold. 1994. *Listen to the Heron's Words: Reimagining Gender and Kinship in North India*. Berkeley: University of California Press.

Roland, Alan. 1988. *In Search of Self in India and Japan: Toward a Cross-Cultural Psychology*. Princeton, NJ: Princeton University Press.

Seymour, Susan. 1993. "Sociocultural Contexts: Examining Sibling Roles in South Asia." In *Siblings in South Asia: Brothers and Sisters in Cultural Context*, ed. Charles Nuckolls, 71–101. New York: Guilford.

Shiva, Vandana. 1989. *Staying Alive: Women, Ecology and Development*. New Delhi: Zed.

Shurmer-Smith, Pamela. 2000. *India: Globalization and Change*. London: Arnold.

Shweder, Richard A. 1991. *Thinking Through Cultures: Expeditions in Cultural Psychology*. Cambridge, MA: Harvard University Press.

Sinha, Jai B.P. 1990. *Work Culture in the Indian Context*. New Delhi: Sage.

Swidler, Ann. 2001. *Talk of Love: How Culture Matters*. Chicago: University of Chicago Press.

Thussu, Daya Kishan. 2000. "The Hinglish Hegemony." In *Television in Contemporary Asia*, ed. David French and Michael Richards, 293–311. New Delhi: Sage.

Vatuk, Sylvia. 1990. "'To Be a Burden on Others': Dependency Anxiety Among the Elderly in India." In *Divine Passions: The Social Construction of Emotion in India*, ed. Owen Lynch, 64–90. Berkeley: University of California Press.

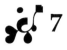 7

WELL-BEING, CULTURAL PATHOLOGY, AND PERSONAL REJUVENATION IN A CHINESE CITY, 1981–2005

William Jankowiak

Introduction

Well-being is a notion that embodies numerous elements ranging from good health to emotional stability to integrated goals for a meaningful life. Life satisfaction is organized around a person's life-orientation or thoughts about the future as they pertain to a person's accomplishments compared to his or her aspirations. Conversely, life dissatisfaction arises whenever an individual's achievements significantly do not match his or her level of aspirations. Given the importance of cultural values in structuring a person's life-orientation or future aspirations, analysis of a culture's notion of well-being needs to explore the interplay between a culture's social organization, its value system, its psychological orientations, and the material opportunities available as they impact a person's life-orientation, and thus the level of aspirations encouraged socially for seeking life satisfaction.

Hollan, in chapter 10, makes an important observation: well-being is an individual affair best understood through probing psychoanalytical investigations. He believes that errors in evaluation arise whenever a psychological phenomenon is extended to a social phenomenon. I partially concur. It is always fruitful to probe an individual's perception of life satisfaction as opposed to globalizing our analysis to include the entire society. This does not mean, however, that we cannot also make society-wide generalizations. Robert Edgerton (1992) suggests there are times when it is appropriate to generalize from the individual condition to include the entire community. This requires a different scale of analysis. He suggests that the levels of health and happiness are two core domains from which to evaluate a society's overall well-being or social fitness. He argues that whenever the majority of people, across all age cohorts, are depressed, malcontent, alienated, fearful, sick, or unable or disinterested in reproducing themselves, the culture can be labeled a "sick society" (Edgerton 1992, 188). I would add to Edgerton's criteria an additional qualification—the scale of societal alienation. Is it a totalizing experience (i.e., extending across most social domains) or is it a more localized experience, felt when an individual enters into a specific domain of interaction? In times of rapid cultural change, there may be a gap between an individual's expectations and accomplishments. In this milieu, personal dissatisfaction is widespread. Correspondingly, there will be certain age cohorts (usually youth) who thrive in the new milieu. In making an assessment of a society's overall well-being, it is necessary first to determine if dissatisfaction is experienced by all or only a few age cohorts. Because rapid social change impacts age cohorts and genders differently, we cannot therefore label an entire culture sick if only people in a few age cohorts are suffering, while people in other age cohorts are thriving. A society in transition may or may not be a "sick society." However, if the majority of people across all age cohorts in a society are miserable, we can infer that the society, at least at that particular moment, is indeed a "sick society."

The "single most common finding from a half century's research," Putnam writes, "is the correlation between life satisfaction and the breadth and depth of one's social connections (Putnam 2000, 385). For Lane (2000), happiness is derived from close bonds of affiliation, which he believes are lacking in the modern world. In contrast, Bell believes that individuals require more than close friendship networks to thrive. Bell writes, "If people have been socialized to participate in a relatively open stratification system, they will seek to establish a set of meanings through which to relate themselves to the wider world" (quoted in Xu 2002, 15). These meanings provide a wider narrative of the good and proper life. Because people need to place themselves within this wider value system, "it should be not only empirically possible, but essential, for most individuals to evaluate their life as a whole" (van Praag and Frijiters 1999, 427).

There is a relationship between the ability to obtain desired goods and services, the freedom to achieve, and well-being (Frey and Stutzer 2002; Inglehart and Klingemann 2000). There is also a strong correlation between well-being and whether or not a society has experienced communist rule (Veenhoven 2000, 282). People everywhere yearn to feel in control of their situations (Anderson 1996; Marmot 2004), I argue; living in a totalitarian social organization will undermine their sense of "being in control" over their immediate environment and, thus, by extension their lives (Langer 1983; Anderson n.d.). This is especially evident for people living in a communist social organization. Freedom House's (1982–1999) studies of well-being in communist societies found that communist political institutions are the worst form of authoritarianism. Life in this political system is experienced with greater "dissatisfaction and suffering than any equivalent social movement in the world's history" (Inglehart and Klingemann 2000, 165–83). People in these societies often suffer from a variety of psychological aliments that arise from the feeling they have no control over their lives (see Courtois et al. 1999 for an historical overview of how people from different societies fared under communism). The importance of control is not confined to people living in industrialized societies. Anthropologists have found that hunter-gatherer and pastoral populations are far more optimistic about their lives than subsistence farming communities, who cannot move if the local ecological conditions worsen and thus are more prone to witchcraft accusations, suspicion, and pessimism about their future (Edgerton 1971).

Sen (2002, 342) stresses (as do ordinary Chinese people I have spoken with) that the two most important qualities for ensuring a good life or well-being are *freedom to choose* and *having the means to obtain desired resources* (i.e., money, land, labor, social networks, and information). Colby (2003, 28) expressed the same notion when identifying autonomy, competence, and affiliation or relatedness as necessary attributes for life satisfaction. Taken together, these perspectives form a kind of self-determination theory of well-being (Ryan and Deci 2000) in which individuals are able to evaluate their lives as ones of satisfaction or dissatisfaction through comparing their goals with their accomplishments, or with the perceived attainability of those goals. From this perspective, well-being is the byproduct of comparing personal accomplishments with aspirations (Frey and Stutzer 2002, 81; Michalos 1991; Inglehart 1990). From this perspective, an individual sense of well-being depends as much upon the possibility of choice and opportunity as it does on the density of one's social connections.

If the freedom to choose is important for personal well-being, what happens when there are drastic restrictions on personal choice? China represents an opportune case to explore this question. Its fifty-plus years of experimenting with a redistributive command economy, combined with periodic bursts of political fever, made extreme egalitarianism more important than other Chinese values recognizing individual merit, vision, and achievement. Throughout much of Chinese history, these values were widely shared, but in the communist era, an alternative cultural model was stressed: social responsibility for the community and nation. Individuals were ideally expected to de-emphasize their individuality in favor of "the common good." In China, the juxtaposition of the two competing value systems—extreme egalitarianism versus individual choice, responsibility, and personal achievement—engendered confusion, anger, angst, and unhappiness. In Maoist China (1949–1976), this accounts, in part, for much of the suffering people experienced in living their lives.

In this paper I examine the Chinese cultural model for life satisfaction or well-being in two different eras: work unit (*danwei*) socialism (1981–83) and market reform (1987, 2000–02). My sample was found in Hohhot, the provincial capital of Inner Mongolia Autonomous Region in northern China, where I lived from 1981–83, for six months in 1987, for five months in 2000, two months in 2002, and one month in 2005, for a total of thirty-nine months. I will examine the ways Chinese sought well-being in four different domains: friendship, family, occupation, and fun activities. By analyzing how Chinese conceptualized their lives over time, I will identify the conceptual frameworks individuals used to assess their relative well-being.

A word on methodology: My initial research was conducted in 1981–83 and again in 1987. In this research, I was not interested in well-being per se. Rather, I focused on seventy-five key families (forty-five Han, thirty Mongol) on a variety of different aspects of their lives, and also visited, observed, and interviewed other residents living throughout the city. The material found in this chapter was taken from my field notes, personal memories of individual lives, and readings in the literature; and although I was not explicitly investigating well-being, concern over well-being is abundantly apparent in the words of the people I interviewed. Because I took field notes on their attitudes toward a host of things in the *danwei* socialist era, I was able to record what Hohhotians actually felt about their lives in the early 1980s and not from what they could later recall about their lives during that era; in this way, I was able to avoid the nostalgia problem apparent, for example, in many of the post–Soviet Union studies, in which there is a clear nostalgia by some for "the good old days" that belies the depth of people's actual dislike for their lives under a communist government. My 2002–05 data was obtained in part through the use of a survey on well-being and happiness given to forty-five Hohhotians (thirty Han and fifteen Mongols; twenty-four females and twenty-one males). Because I did not find ethnicity a factor in well-being, the two groups' responses are combined. I was able to personally interview twenty-nine of the forty-five people surveyed, and thus obtain more in-depth information concerning what they thought about their lives and their future in the market reform era compared with the 1980s. These conversations enabled me to better understand the value Hohhotians placed on social changes. They also enabled me to appreciate the significance of my early 1980s observations.

Self, Family, Morality and Spiritual Well-Being in Chinese History

The theme of self-sufficiency is an important aspect in Chinese spiritual and health practices. The tradition of self-medication and self-sufficiency in healing strived to link the body and the mind together into spiritual wholeness (*yuan*). Qigong masters grounded their teaching in values of "self-control, mastery, assertion, and ... potency" (Chen 2003, 71). The central importance of the interrelationship of body and mind is apparent in the frequency with which bodily metaphors are invoked to convey emotional states (Kleinman 1986).

The foundation of Chinese emotions lies in the corporeal body, with the location of emotions thought to be in the heart (*xin*) (Tung 2000, 78). For most Chinese, affective expressions are intertwined with body idioms, nature metaphors, and ethical codes. Because "the body-person is also the heart-mind's most important single resource" (Elvin 1989, 275), topics of weather, nature, and health often carry within them some evidence of an individual's psychological state. Images of loneliness, for example, may be expressed with reference to isolated clouds or an empty lake or beach.[1] A troubled relationship may be addressed with reference to tumbling leaves along the ground (Tung 2000, 78).

A recurrent theme in classical Chinese writings is the importance of responsibility, choice, and self-growth via achieving mastery of one's body. Contemporary Chinese self-help books focus on developing a nurturing life through moderation, which means consuming the correct food and drink, and maintaining consistency in daily habits.[2] These activities are thought to regulate the heart and mind and, as such, constitute a form of self-improvement (Chen 2003, 263). In this way, Chinese culture has stood against Kierkegaard's and other European existentialist visions that mankind was born to be miserable. For most Chinese, people are born to be happy and content. To achieve this state, however, you need to be proactive in how you live your life.

Chinese philosophical traditions valued reflection, contemplation, independence, responsibility, and achievement. The Confucianists thought that well-being could be achieved through a strict adherence to institutionalized codes of conduct that link role performance to a person's place in the social structure. It is a life orientation consistent with the Confucian emphasis on self-cultivation (Unschuld 1985, 62). In contrast, the Daoists strove to liberate the individual from most social obligations through encouraging individuals to situate themselves within a natural universe. To this end, they stressed conformity and passivity to external forces (Unschuld 1985, 101). Unlike the Confucianists, who associated well-being with proper performance of social rites, the Daoists (much like the Buddhists) linked life satisfaction to a relatively stress-free life best achieved through decreasing one's obligations. This perspective was succinctly summarized in 2002 by a Hohhotian father who advised his twenty-four-year-old son: "Strive to be content and you will find pleasure."

Both philosophical traditions concurred that hard work, self-sufficiency, self-reliance, and self-mastery are essential attributes for having a satisfying life. In time, ordinary Chinese integrated the Confucian and the Daoist cosmologies into a synergetic folk system that continues to guide, at least as an abstraction, their orientation toward how best to live a good life.

The Chinese Communist Vision and the *Danwei* Social Organization

The Communist Party came to power promising to curb governmental complacency, corruption, and economic individualism, and thereby rescue Chinese society from impending economic and moral bankruptcy. Under the party's guidance, a "socialist ethos" was promoted that stressed public virtue over individual gain, the importance of self-denial and social obligations, and an egalitarian lifestyle. This ethos, the party felt, would improve the moral climate and, in turn, increase the productivity of the entire nation. Toward this end, an increased number of "efficient" production and consumption work units (*danwei*) were created to function as combined social, political, and economic institutions by providing, among other things, labor insurance, social security, health benefits, residency and travel permits, as well as serving as a means to administer marriage and divorce and investigate crime (Walder 1986, 28–29; Southall 1993). In effect, enormous resources of power were placed in the hands of the cadre (*ganbu*), a new kind of bureaucrat responsible for the management of the state-sponsored work enterprise.

The Communist Party's authority has been intimately linked to the public's perception that its vision and promise to transform China into a vibrant, modern nation was a worthy aspiration. Critical to the success of the party's political program was the public's continued belief and commitment to that vision. As long as the public as a whole embraced socialism as an ideal and the political elite strove to live according to its professed ideals, the party was honored. The party leaders were, in this era, respected and admired for their integrity and dedication to restoring China's prosperity, a perception that contributed to bolstering the party's political legitimacy.

The Communist Party never questioned the Confucian notion that the best government was staffed by "superior" men (Pye 1985, 41). Unlike their counterparts in Imperial China, the communist elite was not guided by the "wisdom of the classics" but rather by the party doctrine that stressed modesty and unselfish dedication to the collectivity: the nation-state. Nevertheless, the party, much like in Imperial China, reserved its highest esteem for those engaged in public service. Although the party attacked the traditional political and cultural order, it continued to build on the conventional belief that political authority rested on tacit public endorsement. It insisted, therefore, that proper thought, good deeds, and maintaining the highest moral integrity constituted evidence of superiority.

During the initial years of communist rule (1949–54), no one doubted the party's mandate to govern, and there was little disagreement over the cadre's moral and social worth. These shared cultural assumptions engendered public respect and admiration, and, significantly, contributed to promoting China's political unity. The relationship between the cadres and the masses was understood and, for the most part, accepted. Although the party doctrine emphasized the benevolence, dedication, and kindness of its leaders, it was an ideal that was often, in practice, transgressed. However, as long as the public felt that most leaders were dedicated to the public good, and the country's standard of living continued to improve, individual lapses between stated ideals and actual behavior were tolerated if not overlooked.

The enthusiastic support for the Communist Party's socialist vision terminated with the Cultural Revolution (1966–76), marking the end of the public's unquestioned acceptance of the party's political authority. Private and public discourse shifted from unqualified acceptance of the party to a concerted reservation over its political and moral competence. Over time, the party and its membership were increasingly regarded as hypocritical and self-serving. Although the cadre stratum continued to occupy the dominant organizational position (including control of the distribution of resources), it no longer was fully honored.

In the early 1980s, urban China remained organized around a *danwei* (work unit) distribution system that was insular in its orientation and daily policies. It was highly restrictive of individual, social, and geographical mobility. Its opportunity structures were quasi-feudal, with emphasis on political position and bureaucratic rank. The work unit, the local embodiment of the communist state, stressed similar social values to those emphasized in Soviet-dominated Eastern Europe.

In both cultural settings, the good life, as a card (no. 6) in the Czech Communist Museum, Prague puts it, was based on "having a modest income while improving knowledge of the communist doctrines, cooperating with the state bodies, watching cautiously, and being observant as to whether anyone did not disturb the socialist order."

China's *danwei* social insularity fostered a fortress mentality that deemphasized the importance of choice, innovation, and change. Given the difficulty of changing one's employment, people seldom left and seldom did new people arrive. Life was organized around a succession of nonstimulating events and routine social encounters. The *danwei* social organization had a profound numbing effect on the individual's engagement in the wider social universe: with the exception of some intellectuals, the work unit organization restricted one's interest to one's immediate locality. For example, students and teachers at Inner Mongolian University in Hohhot in the 1980s could not imagine crossing the street and visiting the Normal Teachers' College's outstanding library. When I inquired why, everyone acknowledged that unless they knew someone at the Normal College, they would never go to another work unit just to visit. This insularity is evident in the remarks of a young worker who told me in 1983 that he never read the newspaper: "If there is food in the marketplace, I know that everything is fine, and if there is no food, then I know everything is not fine. So, why read the newspaper?"

This parochial outlook was bolstered by limited media outlets as well as by the fact that people seldom traveled. In the 1980s, China's informational technology was seriously undeveloped. For example, there were only two television channels in the city, both with limited program selections. The national news and local weather reports were prerecorded in Beijing and sent the next day via the morning train to Hohhot. This may account for the discrepancy between the weather report and the actual conditions found that day in the city. The work units' structural insularity fostered a nonreflective posture toward the international world. The topic of Taiwanese independence, for instance, was seldom a subject for discussion. People were not, as they are today, emotionally involved with the topic of Taiwan's status. A friend once joked that the local peasants may have heard of Taiwan but did not have a clue as to where it was located. The insularity of ordinary life further contributed to making the extended family the center of social life. Contrary to contemporary American society (Putnam 2000; Lane 2000), people entertained themselves through an endless cycle of visiting among family members and friends. The insularity did not result, however, in the elimination of criticism of the party's policies or the local work unit leader's policy decisions.

Participating in dense friendship networks did not, in and of itself, result in many individuals feeling highly satisfied with their lives. This dissatisfaction arose from the absence of another aspect essential to well-being: the ability to choose and, thus, become responsible for the direction of one's life. In the early 1980s, there was an absence of choice of one's own future goals. This accounts, in large part, for much of the anguish, depression, and ennui so many people felt about life in urban China.

Throughout the early 1980s, Hohhot, like Prague during the Stalinist era, was a "haggard, cold and hungry city where people moved in a gray zone of daily compromise of anger and hidden hopes. … [Within this milieu], there were two essential emotions that characterized the local mentality: melancholy and exaggerated hilarity. The one [was] scarcely conceivable without the other" (Demetz 1997, 322). This mentality is typical of life in totalitarian regimes. Because a totalitarian state "rules by fear … public life becomes brutish" (Brooks 2005, A27); the bonds of civic trust and the normal patterns of social cohesion are undermined, as is public and private morality. The result is that most individual lives are experienced as monotonous and depressing.

In the early 1980s, Chinese urban culture was a storehouse of human wreckage stemming from repeated waves of millennian fervor that left most people completely and totally indifferent to almost anything outside their immediate family's well-being. The dullness of ordinary life was evident in the way people reflected upon their lives. Many Hohhotians tried to survive by being low-keyed in public and focusing on family activities. In 1983, a thirty-four-year-old man matter-of-factly acknowledged his promotion by noting that now, "I may be able to get a new apartment with more rooms [he was living in a one-room apartment]. Maybe become the head of the department in twenty years." He also wanted "to buy a lot of books and book shelves. I want to avoid being sucked into office politics. I want to at least be on a nodding relationship with everyone. In this way, I am protecting myself." After a few moments he added, "I'm rather depressed these days. This life is just not stimulating."

Many Chinese suffered from a kind of spiritual malaise that arose from the perception that they could do nothing to alter their lives' circumstances. This theme was voiced in a twenty-three-year-old male's lamentation: "I lost my dream, I had wanted to study history—Mongolian history. But I can never leave the country. They are afraid of the brain drain. Thus, I cannot go. I must change my plans and become a small businessman." The frustration that grew out of not being in control of one's life can be found in the words of a twenty-seven-year-old married man who, upon learning that his wife's request to transfer to Hohhot had been denied, cried out, "I have no choice, the government controls your life and future." He added, "I hate them all, and want power so that I can hurt others too." A young woman acknowledged that her life was a failure, as she never had an opportunity to pick her job: "I was told to be a clerk. I never had a choice." The yearning of youth to use the full range of their abilities is evident in a letter to the editor published in 1980 in a popular magazine, China Youth (*Zhongguo Qingren*). It reads in part: "Dear Editors: I am twenty-three this year, I should say that I am just beginning life, but already all of life's mystery and charm are gone for me. I feel as if I have reached the end. Looking back on the road I have traveled, I see that I was on a journey from crimson to gray—from hope to disappointment and despair. ... I used to have beautiful illusions about life. ... Now they are all gone." (Xu 2002, 52–53).[3]

People in other age cohorts shared this young woman's negative outlook. A sense of societal anomie can be found in a twenty-nine-year-old mother's reflection on her motivation for having a child: "In China most women have a child because life is so boring that it gives us something to do." Depression is also evident in a fifty-four-year-old government official in his response upon learning that his work unit had given him a bushel of apples: "Yeah, when you get to the middle of the barrel, the rest are all rotten." He added (looking to the ground), "I just go to work and put in the days that follow one after another and life goes on." A fifty-two-year-old man, a minor official, summarized his, and everyone else's exasperation by simply declaring: "I am tired of my life. I want a new life."

I found in my visits to hundreds of families that Hohhotians, regardless of age cohort or gender, spoke in one voice: a general lamentation over the lack of choice, and the boredom and ennui of life. For most, life had become a dead end. The communist social system with its emphasis on rigid egalitarianism, social control, restricted mobility, and conformity undermined many core Chinese cultural values (e.g., achievement, choice, and autonomy). The party's policies were at odds with the Chinese cultural model. In this setting, individuals grew increasingly restless and disappointed with their lives (Jankowiak 1993, 96). If life is about process as much as it is about reaching desired end points, then not being able to choose or seek new avenues heightens senses of personal frustration, and undermines well-being. Because people want a sense of responsibility for how they lead their lives, they "are interested in exploring their personal lives in terms of how they have been able to affect them" (Mines 1988, 576). This pursuit, however, is undermined by the logic of hierarchy that requires complete compliance, with little room left for personal autonomy. Whatever momentary "flow state" (Csikszentmihalyi 1990) or sense of satisfaction urbanites experienced through attending a wedding celebration, participating in an all-night poker event, an evening dance/kissing party, or a Sunday afternoon family dinner, everyone readily acknowledged that when the subject turned to the pursuit of distant goals, they were, by in large, dissatisfied with their lives. Given the presence of a wide sense of alienation that cut across all segments of society, I consider Maoist China to have been a "sick culture."

By 1987, the government's policy toward the market economy was shifting; with it, there was a loss of political control over personal lives. A new, albeit guarded optimism returned to the city. Hohhot, like other Chinese cities, became alive with possibilities. This is not new; for most of Chinese history, there has been a vibrant petty capitalist economy that has stood as an alternative to the tributary state (Gates 1996). Although the *danwei* social structure remained in place, people were aware of an array of opportunities other than those found in state employment. For the first time in Chinese communist history, many college students rejected being assigned a job or "placed" in a rural setting, deciding instead to remain in the city and seek employment in the city's emerging market economy. The increased freedom to pursue personal avenues had an immediate positive impact on Hohhotian's life satisfaction. In 1987, I found that people were noticeably more relaxed and happier about their lives. Their deep-seated cynicism towards communist ideology and restlessness with their life situations had hidden an equally deep-seated idealism and belief in meritocracy, intimacy, friendship ties, and an eagerness to engage life itself; now, for the first time in decades, this could to some extent emerge.

The 1990s Chinese Economic Reforms and the Expansion of Personal Horizons

Tang and Parish's (2000) survey of Chinese urbanites' attitudes toward the future found that in the early 1990s, their overall life satisfaction had declined, especially among educated young men. They also found, however, that positive life satisfaction was associated with the size of the urban setting. The larger the metropolises, Tang and Parish (2000, 120) reported, "the more people were pleased with their life situation and their chances in the reform era." A new ethos that the "the best is yet to come" had emerged. In ensuing years, the newfound hope in the future has been engendered among all but middle-aged laid-off workers (*xiagang*): a sense that the future will bring greater prosperity. China's urban youth expect to do better than their parents in the more challenging local and national marketplace. Moreover, most urbanites believe that China is a rising star in the international community of nations.

If in 1981 Hohhotians spoke of their lost dreams, two decades later my interviewees spoke of dreams they thought could be realized. For them, the future was an array of choices and possibilities. This attitude is captured in a twenty-year-old migrant cook's comment about his dream: "[to] have my own restaurant, [so] that I will be able to travel and go places and learn about the world and become successful in marriage and life. I know that with hard work and dedication I can make it." The young cook's tale is similar to the Horatio Alger stories popular in the United States at the turn of the twentieth century. Alger's heroes were poor boys who faced many challenges before being rewarded with success for their character development and diligence.

Struggle, diligence, and self-mastery continue to be values most Chinese deem essential for the creation of a satisfying life. A twenty-three-year-old youth who moved from a small town to Hohhot said: "I struggle for a better life. It is this struggle to improve that makes life worth living. A kind of faith that I can make it and make life worth living." For him and for most of his friends, he told me, success is not only about obtaining greater material benefits; it is also about the fulfillment of personal goals that are based in mastery of the self. This desire for personal improvement is evident in a thirty-one-year-old female sales clerk who told me: "There are days when I wonder why I could not make a sale—I get depressed. I work very hard. I always wonder how I might improve." It is found in the satisfaction of a thirty-five-year-old mother's reflections on her ten-year-old daughter's future: "I want my child to travel and see the world. I never had the opportunity to travel—I want my child to do this." It is also found in the remarks of a nineteen-year-old man: "I want to embrace and enjoy life as much as I can. I believe in the beauty of life. [I want] to explore the world and dedicate myself to making a difference every day. I want so much to travel around the world." The thrill of involvement is found in a twenty-year-old woman who said: "I was so excited and felt so fulfilled the day I opened my hairdressing salon. ... I knew I was going to learn a lot and improve my position."

The cultural value of self-mastery and personal accomplishment is evident in my 1983 occupational survey, which found that Hohhotians admired people who did things with their lives. Government officials were the least admired and professors (and by association college students) the most admired. My 2000 occupational prestige study found that many Chinese now admired government officials, who were considered to have ability and, to an extent, dedication to their jobs. This shift in sentiment is due, in part, to the professionalization of the bureaucracy, in which more college-educated officials have replaced the "worker-farmer official" who was appointed more for ideological loyalty than for ability.

The ambition to improve oneself, to learn new skills, to be tested in a competitive arena and to succeed, is found in a twenty-four-year-old male who noted: "I could get a good job in Inner Mongolia. ... But in Beijing life is fast. ... I think I can make my fortune in Beijing. I can earn enough to do things, and to get a wife." He added: "I want a challenge. ... Money isn't everything, but it is important these days." For this young man, like so many others I talked to, it was not money per se but the challenge to test his mettle in a major cosmopolitan arena that made Beijing more attractive than Hohhot. The pursuit of self-improvement is found in a twenty-five-year-old man's explanation for quitting his job at a foreign-operated hotel and taking a pay cut in order to take a job that offered better opportunities to learn new tasks, and perhaps personal growth and happiness: "Before, I thought that money was everything. I now realize that there is more to life than consumption and the drive to earn more and more things or find the most beautiful girl."[4]

Rural migrants in Hohhot readily acknowledged that one of the reasons they wanted to live in the city was to train oneself by going through challenging circumstances (*duanlian ziji*), "to open my eyes" (*kaikuo yanjin*) and "to change myself" (*gaibian ziji*) (Zheng 2004, 198; Shanshan Du, email correspondence). In contrast, those who remained in rural areas may feel confined and frustrated over their life circumstances. Rural women may reevaluate their sacrifices for the family well-being; many now wonder if it was worth it. In many ways, the reflections of the rural women who remained behind resemble urbanites of the early 1980s who also complained of boredom, frustration, and unfruitful lives. In both eras, these Chinese have yearned for the freedom to choose, to have opportunities to achieve and to receive respect.

My Hohhot findings are consistent with Fong's (2004) research on Dalian youth attitudes toward the future. Fong discovered that ambitious striving can produce happiness and satisfaction as well as stress and frustration. In effect, achievement and stress are different sides of the same coin (Fong, email correspondence). The dilemma for Chinese youth is to achieve something beyond themselves, while in the process not losing their support network. For most Chinese, life satisfaction arises from mastering both domains.

The Decline of Social Obligations and the Assertion of Self-Interest

In Pushkin's *Eugene Onegin,* one of the central characters says that he can never be happy, since "all we have is duty." This is an attitude that was readily articulated throughout the early 1980s. It is implicit in the popular Chinese expression "it is my duty," voiced whenever I asked someone why he or she helped me. In the 2000–02 field seasons, I did not once hear anyone tell me that they helped me because "it was their duty." The shift from a duty-driven value system to one of personal satisfaction and self-expression is found in a seventeen-year-old woman's observation on why some men sought a young mistress: "If a man is unhappy and desires youth and beauty in another — I can understand why he would want to. ... Happiness is a good motive." The emphasis on personal happiness as a justification constitutes a significant shift in public morality. It is a shift from fulfilling social conventions to following one's own inner prompting. In effect, urban China is witnessing the emergence of an emotive ethos that justifies personal authenticity as much as social obligation.

In the 1980s there was a cultural consensus as to where one should be in the life cycle in order to accomplish certain things. It is clear that China's younger generation no longer hold to those ideas, and when they do, it is not as strong as it was for their parents. The cultural norms have shifted to allow for greater individual discretion, not least in terms of mate selection criteria. A twenty-three-year-old woman's description of her ideal mate is representative of the replacement of instrumental considerations (e.g., income, connections) with those that value personality, compatibility, and character development. She yearned for "a man who I can explore and share feelings with and experience the beauty of life. I want to accept him as himself, and to learn to appreciate one another and what we have to offer one another." Both men and women emphasized their development as unique individuals, free from customary obligations. This point reverberated in a twenty-four-year-old man's reflections on why he broke up with his girlfriend: "She was so forceful, and I felt I could not develop myself; I could not express myself." A twenty-three-year-old woman's criterion for her ideal husband or boyfriend is based just as much on psychological attributes as it is on material possessions: "I want a man who is committed to a cause, something larger than himself. I want a man who is internally motivated."

Before the 1990s, a job was little more than a statement of one's position within the *danwei* organizational hierarchy that prioritized social rank over all else. In the new urban market economy, there are more possibilities to discover a viable niche that may result in individual fulfillment. In effect, work now holds the possibility for personal growth and with it, new avenues in which to obtain self-respect. In the early 1980s, life goals and job satisfaction were seldom linked. No one discussed the importance of job or career; most people stressed the importance of their hobbies. Moreover, people noted that the workplace was a center of suspicion and ill will. In contrast, by 2000, many urbanites noted how much they liked to be engaged in work. A twenty-four-year-old woman said that she "loves working—when I wake up and have nothing to do, I panic and make up tasks." A thirty-seven-year-old man acknowledged that "in the past, no one liked to work. The official (*ganbu*) had the power—you gave gifts to him. The work was not interesting and you received no benefits for innovation. Now, more and more people like their jobs, but maybe not their salary! People like choice and the freedom to leave. The fact that bosses reward your good work with bonuses is also a plus." Unlike in the 1980s, job mobility is a constant in urban China, as evidenced by the frequency of urban job fairs organized to attract potential employees, many of whom are currently working at rival companies.

When Chinese men and women discuss the importance of choice, achievement, and self-mastery, there is little variation in their response. Whenever I asked about happy times, people provided concrete examples: chatting with friends, playing with their child, having dinner with the family, visiting grandparents (who raised them). But when asked about the future, people invoked more abstract principles of self-cultivation, achievement, and self-mastery. In my 2002 survey, I found that young men and women's values as compared to their parents' generation were focused more on self expression and fulfillment than on role obligations and proper performance. For urban youth, ego fulfillment has become the predominate metaphor in which to evaluate their lives. There are, however, gender differences in perceptions of well-being. These are evident when men and women discuss the importance of family life, children, and marriage. Most married women stressed a balance in the way they weighed their relationship with their family and husband. Middle-aged women, in particular, noted the importance of sacrifice, a value seldom voiced by their offspring. Women continued to stress the importance of their natal family, their child, and, if not married, their boyfriend. Upon becoming a mother, most women gave more emphasis to the parent-child relationship than their relationship with their husband. For example, a thirty-three-year-old married woman said, "I worry about my children. Will they be able to eat well? If my business is not good, I can't afford tuition and related expenses. I am less concerned with myself, but I am very concerned about them." In a way, many women felt empowered by their decision to seek fulfillment in the conventional role of motherhood.

In both eras (1980–2000), men stressed the importance of obtaining recognition, respect, and earning money, necessary for the achievement of success. For men, emotional intimacy with their wives, at least at the level of an abstraction, was an important value, whereas for most women, childbirth alters their value priorities in favor of their natal family and only child. For married women, their relationship with their husband is a secondary consideration. Nonetheless, both sexes' dreams of the future are remarkably similar. Both wanted to travel, sightsee, learn new things, and have enough money to do the things they want to do.

Conclusion

It is well known, though not entirely accepted, that the communist movements in China, the Soviet Union, and elsewhere have produced in their wake more unhappiness and greater dissatisfaction that any similar type of movement in human history (Courtois et al. 1999). The study of well-being in China provides a framework for understanding why the communist social movement brought so much misery in its wake. People desire a sense of control over their lives in terms of freedom of movement, and the ability to participate in activities that bring a sense of accomplishment. Indeed, Marmot's (2004) extensive review of the literature found that when people have control over their environment, it improves their overall health and well-being.

Governments that experiment with promoting happiness, Popper writes (1963, 227), are very likely to want to control the circumstances of people's lives in order to make their experiments pay off. This was especially so for Maoist China. The Communist Party's emphasis on heavy industry combined with the leveling policies of the Cultural Revolution destroyed mobility opportunities for most people (Tang and Parish 2000, 310). In effect, state policy instituted a series of social changes that disrupted the fit between cultural understanding and opportunity (see Derné's chapter 6 for an excellent discussion of this relationship). Following Mao's death in 1976, there was a loosening of some of the authoritarian policies, encouraging many people to reconsider their life opportunities. But the work unit system remained in place, which heightened individual frustration, anger, and a sense of alienation in people's lives.

Western societies are often characterized as providing an abundance of opportunities, but at the cost of a reduction in social connections (Lane 2000). In contrast, in China throughout the early 1980s, there were abundant personal connections but few opportunities for achievement. Consequently, Hohhotians sought fulfillment in family matters, in marriage, having a child, and in friendship. By the mid-1990s, most Hohhotians wanted other things: for some, family, for others, a fulfilling career and adventure, and for still others, a dream to be fulfilled. Urban Chinese yearned for something more than endless days of congeniality. What many now want is the opportunity to become involved with a wider social universe of possibilities. In effect, they want the opportunity to become responsible for their individual life careers. This does not mean that Hohhotians or other Chinese cannot find deep satisfaction in fulfilling social obligations or seeking emotional fulfillment through family or community connections. Clearly, many can and do. What is critical for personal well-being is that an individual believes that it was his or her own choice to engage life in a given fashion.

While choice is essential to well-being, greater choice does not necessarily mean greater well-being. Rather, well-being is a combination of aspirations and the presence of opportunities to achieve them. Its existence, combined with economic growth, provides people with the material and spiritual sense that life is getting better. Throughout the 1980s, urban China was organized around compliance and not individual choice. By the later 1990s, except for laid-off workers (*xiagang*) and others without economic opportunities, most urban Chinese felt better about their life situations, and, thus, their personal lives. Tangible opportunities are just as important as the ability to strive for personal well-being. In the end, the achievability of one's aspirations is as important as having the freedom to choose these aspirations.

At the start of the twenty-first century, China, much like the United States in the 1950s, has an economy that is expanding, as are its national hopes and aspirations. It is an optimistic moment. People are happy about their prospects. From an analytical point of view, Western-trained social scientists see the emergence in the new China of stark inequalities and widening social disparities between various segments of society, while ordinary Chinese continue to see opportunities and choices, and feel a heightened sense of well-being in their lives. It remains to be seen how the Chinese will feel when the inevitable downturn in the economy restricts opportunity and with it the assumption of unlimited possibilities. For now, most Chinese have a heightened sense of well-being and are glad to have the opportunity to scheme, speculate, and place their lives into what many believe is a horizon of unlimited possibilities.

Notes

I would like to thank Gene Anderson, Dan Benyshek, Nick Colby, Steve Derné, Stacy Garreston, Helen Gerth, Vanessa Fong, Libby Hinson, Lisa Hoff, Carolina Izquierdo, Gordon Mathews, Stanley Rosen, and Geeta Tiwari for their encouragement, insights, and thoughtful remarks.

1. As Tung (2000) observed, the Chinese do not say "peace of mind." They say "peace of heart." Mood is *xin jin,* "territory of the heart," and sorrow is *shang xin,* "the heart is wounded." To long for someone dearly, especially a child, is often expressed as *xin tong,* "the heart is aching" (over the child). The same term also refers to bodily sensation, as in chest pain. "To know a person's heart is to know the entire person" (Tung 1994, 486).
2. The Chinese have always been obsessed with the physical side of the human body as a means of preserving longevity. It is believed that through practices such as *taiji, qigong,* herbal tonics, fan dancing, year-round swimming, dancing, mountain climbing, and bedroom arts, disease can be kept away and a pleasurable, comforting and stable body can be produced (Farquhar 2002, 262).
3. Her sentiment is remarkably similar to what Chinese had experienced forty-odd years earlier on the eve of the 1938 Japanese invasion of Beijing (then Peiping). A Chinese servant recalls that "there is something worse than physical destruction. The oppression and control which are more terrible for a people than rape and murder and opium addiction" (Pruitt 1945, 3).
4. The situation for Mongols has been somewhat different than that of the Chinese. In the 1980s, Mongols had high expectations about the government's minority policy, and were optimistic about the future. The post-Tiananmen years have seen an increase in police presence and more arrests of urban Mongols. Consequently, urban Mongols tend to be more dissatisfied than I remember in conversations with them in the 1980s, when they hoped the government would adjust its minority policies and respond to their concerns. When the topic shifted to other domains, however, Mongols' levels of satisfaction reflected their Han counterparts. It was only in the arena of ethnic policy that they were noticeably less satisfied.

References

Anderson, Eugene. 1996. *Ecologies of the Heart.* New York: Oxford University Press.
———. n.d. *Floating World Lost.* Manuscript.
Brooks, David. 2005. "Mourning Mother Russia." *New York Times,* May 23, A27.
Chen, Nancy. 2003. *Breathing Spaces: Qigong, Psychiatry, and Healing in China.* New York: Columbia University Press.
Colby, Benjamin N. 2003. "Toward a Theory of Culture and Adaptive Potential." *Human Complex Systems. Mathematical Anthropology and Culture Theory: An International Journal* 1 (3): 1–53.

Courtois, Stéphane, et al. 1999. *The Black Book of Communism*. Cambridge: Cambridge University Press.

Csikszentmihalyi, Mihaly. 1990. *Flow: The Psychology of Optimal Experience*. New York: Harper Perennial.

Demetz, Peter. 1997. *Prague in Black and Gold: Scenes from the Life of a European City*. New York: Hill and Wang.

Diener, Ed and Eunkook M. Suh, eds. 2000. *Culture and Subjective Well-Being*. Cambridge, MA: MIT Press.

Edgerton, Robert. 1971. *The Individual in Cultural Adaptation: A Study of Four East African Peoples*. Berkeley: University of California Press.

———. 1992. *Sick Societies*. New York: Free Press.

Elvin, M. 1989. "Tales of Shen and Xin: Body Person and Heart Mind in China during the last 150 years." *Fragments for a History of the Human Body*, ed. M. Feher, part 2, 267–349. New York: Zone.

Farquhar, Judith. 2002. *Appetites*. Durham, NC: Duke University Press.

Fong, Vanessa L. 2004. *Only Hope: Coming of Age Under China's One-Child Policy*. Stanford, CA: Stanford University Press.

Freedom House. 1982–1999. *Freedom in the World: The Annual Survey of Political Rights and Civil Liberties*. New York.

Frey, Bruno and Alois Stutzer. 2002. *Happiness and Economics*. Princeton, NJ: Princeton University Press.

Gates, Hill. 1996. *China's Motor: A Thousand Years of Petty Capitalism*. New York: Cornell University Press.

Inglehart, Ronald. 1990. *Culture Shift in Advanced Industrial Society*. Princeton, NJ: Princeton University Press.

Inglehart, Robert and Hans Dieter Klingemann. 2000. "Genes, Culture, Democracy and Happiness." In *Culture and Subjective Well-Being*, ed. Ed Diener and Eunkook M. Suh, 165–83. Cambridge, MA: MIT Press.

Jankowiak, William. 1993. *Sex, Death, and Hierarchy in a Chinese City*. New York: Columbia University Press.

Kleinman, Arthur. 1986. *Social Origins of Distress and Disease: Depression, Neurasthenia, and Pain in Modern China*. New Haven, CT: Yale University Press.

Lane, Robert. 2000. *The Loss of Happiness in Market Democracies*. New Haven, CT: Yale University Press.

Langer, Ellen J. 1983. *The Psychology of Control*. Beverly Hills, CA: Sage.

Marmot, Michael. 2004. *The Status Syndrome: How Social Standing Affects Our Health and Longevity*. New York: Times Book/Henry Holt.

Michalos, Alex. 1991. "Global Report on Student Well-Being." Vol. 1. *Life Satisfaction and Happiness*. New York: Springer.

Mines, Mattison. 1988. "Conceptualizing the Person: Hierarchical Society and Individual Autonomy in India." *American Anthropologist* 90 (3): 568–79.

Popper, Karl. 1963. *The Open Society and its Enemies*. Princeton: Princeton University Press.

Pruitt, Ira. 1945. *The Daughter of Han*. Stanford, CA: Stanford University Press.

Putnam, Robert. 2000. *Bowling Alone: The Collapse and Revival of American Community*. New York: Simon and Schuster.

Pye, Lucian. 1985. *Asian Power and Politics*. Cambridge, MA: Harvard University Press.

Ryan, Robert and E. Deci. 2000. "Self-determination Theory and the Facilitation of Intrinsic Motivation, Social Development, and Well-Being." *American Psychologist* 55 (1): 68–78.

Sen, Amartya. 2002. *Rationality and Freedom*. Cambridge, MA: Belknap Press.

Southall, Aidan. 2000. *The City in Time and Space*. New York: Cambridge University Press.

Suh, Eunkook M. 2000. "Self, the Hyphen Between Culture and Subjective Well-Being." In *Culture and Subjective Well-Being*, ed. Ed Diener and Eunkook M. Suh, 63–86. Cambridge, MA: MIT Press.

Tang, Wenfang and William Parish. 2000. *Chinese Urban Life Under Reform: The Changing Social Contract*. Cambridge: Cambridge University Press.

Tung, May Pao-may. 1994. "Symbolic Meanings of the Body in Chinese Culture and 'Somatization.'" *Culture, Medicine, and Psychiatry* 18: 483–92.

———. 2000. *Chinese Americans and Their Immigrant Parents*. New York: Haworth Clinical Practice Press.

Unschuld, Paul. 1985. *Medicine in China: A History of Ideas*. Berkeley: University California Press.

Van Praag, Bernard and Paul Frijters. 1999. "The Measurement of Welfare and Well-Being: The Leyden Approach." In *Well-Being: The Foundations of Hedonic Psychology*, ed. Daniel Kahnemann, Ed Diener, and Norbert Schwarz, 413–33. New York: Russell Sage Foundation.

Veenhoven, Ruut. 2000. "Freedom and Happiness." In *Culture and Subjective Well-Being*, ed. Ed Diener and Eunkook M. Suh, 257–88. Cambridge, MA: MIT Press.

Walder, Andrew G. 1986. *Communist Neo-Traditionalism: Work and Authority in Chinese Industry*. Berkeley: University of California Press.

Xu, Luo. 2002. *Searching For Life Meaning: Changes and Tensions in the World Views of Chinese Youth in the 1980's*. Ann Arbor: The University of Michigan Press.

Zheng, Tian. 2004. "From Peasant Women to Bar Hostesses: Gender and Modernity in Post-Mao Dalian." In *On the Move: Women and Rural-to-Urban Migration in Contemporary China*, ed. Arianne M. Gaetano and Tamara Jacka, 80–108. New York: Columbia University Press.

8

FINDING AND KEEPING A PURPOSE IN LIFE
Well-Being and *Ikigai* in Japan and Elsewhere
Gordon Mathews

Well-being is not only a matter of physical health; it has an existential component as well. In order to fully experience well-being, people everywhere need to feel that their lives are worth living. This sense is difficult to specify in most languages, because there is no term for it. However, Japanese has exactly such a term: *ikigai,* meaning "that which most makes one's life worth living," whether one's work, family, dream, or God. I argue that once we move beyond the barrier of language—the lack of a term like *ikigai* in languages other than Japanese—the same is the case for people in societies beyond Japan. When Americans, for example, say things like, "Do you *really* love me?" or "My kids mean everything to me," they too are talking about *ikigai,* even if they lack a word for it.

This chapter begins by examining the place of "what makes life worth living" in analyses of well-being, and discusses the methodological problems inherent in such analysis. It then considers the complex meanings and usages of *ikigai* in Japan today. Subsequently, it offers a more abstract conception of *ikigai,* enabling us to consider the application of *ikigai* to societies beyond Japan. *Ikigai,* this chapter argues, may serve as a way to compare individuals in different societies in the cultural formulation, social negotiation, and institutional channeling of their senses of what makes their lives worth living. On this basis, this paper compares *ikigai* in Japan, the United States, and Hong Kong to illustrate one way in which *ikigai*—and perhaps well-being—may be comprehended cross-culturally.

Ikigai and Well-Being

In order to fully understand well-being in different societies, I maintain that we must consider the existential dimension of our lives. We need to consider this dimension because a person can have good physical health, live in a humane and just society, be financially well off, and have reasonably good human relationships, and yet still not experience a sense of well-being. Numerous works of contemporary fiction by authors from John Updike to Milan Kundera to Haruki Murakami show how even those who live comfortable lives in affluent societies may find their lives to be fundamentally unfulfilling. Something more is required for well-being. That "something more" is a sense of the purpose and significance of one's life.

The pursuit of significance is universal (Becker 1971, 1974), but the forms and styles through which a sense of significance is pursued vary dramatically in different societies, just as they vary among individuals. The devout Muslim in Pakistan, like the evangelical Christian in the United States, may pursue significance primarily through a relationship with the divine. The Chinese or American patriot may pursue significance in terms of love for one's country. The Japanese or French company worker may find significance in work, albeit in different institutionally and culturally shaped ways, just as Chinese parents may find significance through their children in a somewhat different idiom than German or Mexican parents. The dream of romantic love serves as a promise of significance for many; and dropouts and mavericks in a range of societies may locate their pursuit of significance in creative activity or travel or spiritual pursuits. People in tribal or agricultural societies located significance in forms that we can now scarcely comprehend except through an effort of imagination, as ethnographic life histories attest.[1] But the pursuit of significance itself is a matter of being human.

A major problem confronted by the investigator is one of how this pursuit of significance can be explored. Most people are not fully conscious of how they pursue significance, since it is part of their most intimate inner experience; so how can the investigator discover this? Aside from the standard difficulties of interviewing—how much the person one interviews is consciously concealing information, and so on—there is also the underlying problem of getting at an area of experience that the interviewee may never have articulated, and thus the danger that their expressed words may fail to fully reflect their inner experience.

This is a problem not just for this chapter, but for the anthropological study of well-being in general. How can we understand another person's sense of well-being? We can ask a person "How do you feel about your life?" in different ways, but we cannot understand how they actually experience their lives. There is a gap between experience and expression, worlds and words; the anthropologist can talk to interviewees, but cannot enter their minds, to experience the world as they do.

Anthropologists may compare *conceptions* of well-being across cultures, but cannot easily compare the *experience* of well-being. In one anthropologist's cautionary words, "While public, shared concepts must help to shape private experience, it remains doubtful whether anthropologists have means for gaining access to that experience as experience" (Harris 1989, 601–2).[2] Many of the chapters in this book sidestep this by exploring cultural conceptions of well-being as much as actual experiences of well-being. But it must be remembered that this is not the study of well-being as actually experienced, which remains inevitably elusive, but rather of the cultural frameworks within which well-being is conceived of and expressed.

My own research has fallen within this limitation (Mathews 1996). But I maintain that by exploring individuals' pursuit of significance not as a psychological matter within individuals' minds, but as a sociological and anthropological matter of individuals' social linkages, the difficulties inherent in attempting to understand the pursuit of significance can be mitigated. Anthropology's specialty is considering how the mind is culturally shaped by and shaping of its social world. *Ikigai* can serve as a means for such understanding; it can provide a window into how well-being is culturally, socially, and institutionally shaped in different societies. *Ikigai* in Japanese is a complex term, with two major meanings (Kamiya 1980, 15; Kobayashi 1989, 25). One meaning is "the feeling that one's life is worth living" (*ikigai-kan*). *Ikigai* in this sense seems close to the subjective sense of "well-being." *Ikigai* has, however, another meaning; it is also "the object [the entity in the world] that makes one's life worth living" (*ikigai taishō*), whether one's work, one's lover, one's children, one's dream, or one's God. *Ikigai* in this sense is not "well-being" as experienced—which, I argue (in contrast to Hollan, chapter 10), remains largely impenetrable to the anthropological analyst—but that element of one's social world that enables one to experience well-being. It is in this sense that I believe *ikigai* to be analyzable and cross-culturally comparable. This analysis will require removing the concept of *ikigai* from its Japanese cultural moorings, to define it in a more abstract cross-cultural form. Before we proceed to that, however, let me provide a brief portrait of the complexities of *ikigai* as a cultural concept in Japan today.

Ikigai in Its Japanese Cultural Context

I first went to Japan in 1980; I still remember being amazed to find that the Japanese language had a term such as *ikigai,* and that Japanese people might talk in their daily lives about what made their lives worth living. The term *ikigai* is commonly used in Japan; one hears statements such as "my *ikigai* is my family," "my *ikigai* is mountain climbing," and "my *ikigai* is to serve the public in volunteer activity." Mass media in Japan regularly comment on *ikigai*; popular books discuss "how to find *ikigai* after you retire" (Kanamaru 1999), "how to educate students so that they can find *ikigai*" (Iida 2004), and "how adults with mental disabilities can feel *ikigai*" (Shiraishi 1998), among many other topics. Newspaper articles as well as scholarly books offer *ikigai* surveys showing, for example, that "21 percent of company workers find their *ikigai* in work," or "34 percent of mothers find *ikigai* in their children" (see, to take one example of such surveys, Mita 1984, 59–66). These statistical measures, whatever their validity, show that *ikigai* as what one lives for is a commonly accepted term in Japan today.

Despite this, however, *ikigai* is difficult to fully grasp for many Japanese. This is partly because it is an abstraction. The Japanese-language Google search engine, when queried as to *ikigai,* comes up with 750,000 hits; a search of Japanese-language Amazon.com shows some two hundred book titles bearing the word. But a closer examination of these books and websites reveals that many use *ikigai* in their titles, but do not discuss *ikigai* at all in their content, where the word may not even appear. The term *ikigai* is clearly attractive to writers and readers; but in these forums, its meaning is often left unspecified, referring to happiness, fulfillment, or other broad concepts.

Ikigai has been difficult to grasp because it is abstract, but also because its meanings have been contested. In the 1970s and 1980s (Mathews 1996, 12–26), *ikigai* was formulated in different books and articles in different ways. In some, it was treated as "self-realization" (*jiko jitsugen*) (Kobayashi 1989) and in others as "commitment to one's group" (*ittaikan*) (Niwano 1969).[3] These different formulations have different practical meanings. If (to follow the standard Japanese gender-role division of that era, if less so today) a man finds *ikigai* in work, this may be because of his commitment to his company and corporate role (*ittaikan*) or alternatively, because of the individual fulfillment he finds in work (*jiko jitsugen*); if a woman finds *ikigai* in family, it may be because of her commitment to the role of wife and mother (*ittaikan*) or because of the individual fulfillment she feels from her family (*jiko jitsugen*). If *ikigai* is seen as self-realization, then if work or family isn't fulfilling, one may feel justified in leaving; but if *ikigai* is a matter of commitment to a group, then leaving is no more than selfishness, an abrogation of one's deepest commitment. I postulated (1996, 26) that while *ikigai* in print media was shifting in its dominant meaning from "commitment to group" to "self-realization," what this meant in Japanese life at large was unclear. Was *ikigai* as "self-realization" the Japanese future, or was it an ongoing unattainable dream for most Japanese, making bearable a constraining reality based on "commitment to group"?

This is still unclear a decade or more later. Today, living for one's own fulfillment has become the dominant cultural meaning of *ikigai* in Japan, but this is still not an accepted norm in Japanese institutions. Over the past fifteen years, the Japanese institutional order has lost considerable credibility. Economic doldrums have eroded the ideal of "living for one's company," with "lifetime employment" having been shaken although not yet discarded (*Economist* 2005, 4). Despite this, many Japanese companies continue to be structured so as to demand total commitment from their regular (male) employees, just as many Japanese schools and childcare facilities continue to be structured so as to demand total commitment of mother to child. In this sense, *ikigai* as commitment to group and role continues, as institutionally mandated if not culturally supported—if you are a regular company employee or a mother, you may find yourself with little choice but to live as if commitment to these roles was your *ikigai*.

A remarkable change in recent years has been that increasing numbers of young people choose (or are forced by the lack of available career-track jobs) not to enter the career-track employment path of their fathers but to instead become temporary employees (*furiitaa*), operating cash registers for convenience stores while dreaming of futures as fashion designers or rock musicians or internet journalists (*Furiitaa kenkyūkai* 2001; Mathews 2004). They thus reject the *ikigai* of work and company, to find it in their dreams instead.[4] At the same time, increasing numbers of young people choose not to marry but to stay home and live with their parents as "parasite singles" (M. Yamada 1999; Nakano and Wagatsuma 2004), while pursuing *ikigai* as career dream or play; they thus reject *ikigai* as family. These young people—perhaps as many as 30 or even 40 percent of Japanese aged twenty-four to forty, although accurate statistics seem impossible to come by—represent a rejection of the "commitment to group and role" held as de facto *ikigai* by many of their parents.

This is a dominant shift in *ikigai* that I have seen in Japanese society over the past decade—millions of young people refusing to follow the *ikigai* paths of their parents—but while the emergence of these young people has garnered much media attention, it is not much discussed in books and web sites on *ikigai*. A predominant focus in these books and web sites is not the young who refuse to give up their dreams to live for work or family, but rather the old, those who have lived for work or family but now find themselves adrift. This reflects another trend in Japanese society: the increasing numbers of elderly in a society with one of the longest life expectancies in the world. These are the men and women who in earlier decades lived for company or family, but who now find that they have shed these roles and require something new to live for; their earlier commitment to group has left many of them ill-prepared for a life outside such groups. There are hundreds of municipalities today that advertise *"ikigai* centers" for elders, where old people can mingle with their friends and pursue various activities, as well as perhaps engage in volunteer work.

The problem of the elderly finding a purpose to live for, as well as that of the young refusing to adapt to "adult society," is in its particulars unique to Japan. Few developed societies have an adult social order demanding such suppression of self for the sake of role. Many young people seek not to join that order, and many elders feel lost once they leave that order, having no selves left to which to return. However, the problems of a "generation gap" felt by many youth, and of increasing numbers of elderly cast off by society, obviously transcend Japan. These are problems faced, more or less, by societies the world over.

The global reach of *ikigai* problems today is prefigured by the historical evolution of the term. We have seen how *ikigai* in the 1970s and 1980s was conceived of in two ways, as self-realization and as commitment to one's group. This is an echo of the historical transformation of the term (Wada 2001, 28–32), from its earlier formulation as fulfilling socially recognized values and roles to its later formulation as fulfilling one's own individual purpose in life. According to Wada, this transformation in the meaning of *ikigai* took place in the Meiji era (1867–1912), although both meanings have continued to be used. It is perhaps no coincidence that the Meiji era paralleled the years during which European analysts began pondering the meanings of society's newly emergent individualism, leading Durkheim to write of "the cult of the individual" and the moral reconstitution of society in the modern age (Marske 1987), and Weber to ask "What motives determine and lead the individual members [of communal society] ... to behave in such a way that the community ... continues to exist?" (Weber 1964 [1925], 107). This conjunction of concerns over individualism implies that the reformulation of *ikigai* in Japan was not a matter for Japan alone, but rather a Japanese reflection of global modernity. This in turn indicates that *ikigai* and its analysis transcends Japan, as we will now explore.

Ikigai Considered Cross-culturally

The term *ikigai,* in all its nuances, apparently only exists in Japan. There is a similar term in Korean, but it does not have the everyday salience that *ikigai* has in Japanese (Mori 1999), and is apparently not often used. French terms such as *joie de vivre* and *raison d'être* also bear a similarity to the two different meanings of *ikigai,* but are more philosophical in nuance than *ikigai* (Kamiya 1980, 14–15). There is no clear answer to why *ikigai* as an everyday term apparently exists in Japan alone, among all the societies in which it might have appeared, but the historical circumstances mentioned above—the change in meaning of *ikigai*—imply historical happenstance. Japanese had a convenient word in waiting that could be shifted in its meaning to specify the individuation of onrushing modernity, as other societies did not.

In any case, the concept of *ikigai* appears cross-cultural in its validity. Japanese scholars are examining *ikigai* across the globe (Takahashi and Wada 2001). While these efforts are flawed by the lack of a common definition of *ikigai,* they do reveal Japanese scholars' convictions that *ikigai* is comparable cross-culturally: it is not a term whose meanings apply to Japan alone. I myself have explored (Mathews 1996) how *ikigai* can be used to compare Japanese and Americans as to how they pursue lives worth living. On this basis, it seems possible to formulate a cross-cultural definition of *ikigai.* I argue that *ikigai* may be conceptualized not simply as "that which makes one's life worth living," but also as "one's deepest bond to one's social world"/"one's deepest sense of social commitment." *Ikigai* may serve as a way to compare individuals in different societies as to how they are linked to their societies.

There are significant methodological problems apparent in using *ikigai* as a cross-cultural variable. Does everyone have an *ikigai*? Most adults in affluent societies apparently do, in that some aspect of their lives makes their lives as a whole seem worth living to them, or so my own and others' research has indicated (Mathews 1996; Takahashi and Wada 2001, 160–214); but people can live without *ikigai,* although not happily. Do people have just one *ikigai,* or can they have several? Some people do indeed seem to have a balance of different *ikigai;* but often, once a series of dilemmas are set before them, a single *ikigai* emerges. To what extent does *ikigai* change? *Ikigai* usually changes over the life course, for example, when one falls in love, has children, or retires; but it is relatively stable. The majority of people locate *ikigai* in their future dreams when young, and in work or family in their prime of life; sustaining these *ikigai* may become problematic in old age. What is the relation of *ikigai* to well-being? *Ikigai* is undoubtedly a major factor in well-being—arguably one cannot attain a state of well-being without *ikigai*—but the terms are not synonymous. These definitional uncertainties are very real, but do not mitigate the value of *ikigai* as an analytical tool, as I hope the remainder of this chapter will show.

We can analyze *ikigai* cross-culturally in terms of the following statement:

> On the basis of culturally and personally shaped fate, individuals strategically formulate and interpret their *ikigai* from an array of cultural conceptions, negotiate these *ikigai* within their circles of immediate others, and pursue their *ikigai* as channeled by their society's institutional structures so as to attain and maintain a sense of the personal significance of their lives (Mathews 1996, 49–50).

Let me elaborate. We are shaped by culturally and personally shaped fate. We are born into a particular society and family that shapes us before we have any comprehension of what is happening; we emerge as volitional beings having been shaped by a fate over which we have had no control or even awareness. Beyond this, as we grow older, we become products of our own biography, which we cannot ever fully escape. This inevitably shapes how we conceive of and pursue *ikigai*.

We strategically formulate *ikigai* in that we interpret what we live for through our use of cultural conceptions. We in the developed world increasingly live within a global "cultural supermarket" (Mathews 2000); every library and every internet link provide an array of potential *ikigai* formulations. However, our society promulgates some ideas more than others: public schooling and television delimit the cultural supermarket, making some ideas seem far more palatable and "natural" than others. Not everyone follows these dominant ideas, but most people do.

We do so because all cultural formulations of *ikigai* must be socially negotiated, and the social world is narrower than the cultural world. We socially negotiate *ikigai* with our immediate others—spouse, children, coworkers, friends—in terms of how we define our deepest senses of commitment vis-à-vis those others, who are in competition to be the object of our deepest commitment. This *ikigai* competition may be seen daily, in mundane conversations that may not appear to be about *ikigai*, but in fact are: "Do you love me?" "Of course I love you!" ["Am I your *ikigai*?" "Of course you are! (But I'm not allowed to answer in any other way. ...)]" "Going home early again today?" ["I make this work my *ikigai*! Why don't you? What the hell's wrong with you?"] "Honey, I'm really sorry, but I've got extra work: I can't come home until late tonight." "But you promised! It's your daughter's birthday!" ["Which is your real *ikigai,* your work or your family?" "For now, anyway, it's my work."]. Multiple entities in our lives want us to live for them. Because we each live within multiple social worlds, we experience this competition in our lives, at least until these entities make a truce with one another, as they often do.

Ikigai is channeled by institutional structures, in that the structural principles organizing a society encourage or necessitate the pursuit of one's deepest commitment down some paths and not down others. This institutional channeling may be coercive, as when young men may be required to "die for their country." More typically, it "encourages" the individual down one *ikigai* path instead of another by, for example, making higher education the prerequisite for high-paying positions, or by providing or not providing institutionalized childcare or social security. These institutional policies may have decisive effects on the individual's pursuit of *ikigai*—whether a young person should bother with university as a path to fulfilling her dream, whether a woman should pursue a career or stay at home raising children, or whether a middle-aged person should take a risk in her career.

Finally, the self attains a sense of personal significance through *ikigai.* The pursuit of significance is the existential meaning of *ikigai;* as individuals we seek to matter beyond ourselves, and *ikigai* can enable us to matter, by profoundly linking us to the social world, the source of meaning in our lives, as Durkheim pointed out (1965 [1915]). Paradoxically, *ikigai* is also profoundly individual: although institutional structures of society may channel *ikigai* down certain paths, and pressure from others may nudge the pursuit of *ikigai* down some paths and not others, *ikigai* is something that no one outside oneself can fully mandate.

In 1989–1991, I interviewed (Mathews 1996) 102 Japanese and Americans, asking them about work, family, and friends; the story of their lives up to the present; and their dreams, hopes, fears, and religious beliefs. These interviews took place over two to four meetings over four to ten hours. Only after our discussions were almost completed did I broach *ikigai,* asking, "What's most important to you in your life? What's your *ikigai*? and sometimes, "After all you've told me, it seems that XXX is most important in your life/your *ikigai.* Does that seem accurate to you?" In this way, I could avoid abstract philosophizing and could tie what the people specifically described about their lives to their *ikigai.* In the years since these interviews, I have conducted follow-up interviews with some of these people, and my students and I have collected a broad range of interviews with Hong Kongers as well: 84 interviews in all. These have been shorter, two to three hours over one to two meetings, but have followed the same interview sequence.

Such interviewing is not without problems: there is an inevitable gap between what the people we interviewed tell us, and how they actually live their lives.[5] Nonetheless, I argue that this is the best that can be achieved, given the fact that I cannot live with these people for months on end, to see the inevitable contradictions in their lives; I have little choice but to base my analysis of their lives of what they say, at length. In this chapter, rather than discuss individuals in their pursuit of *ikigai,* I turn, on the basis of the interviews conducted in three societies, to the comparison of societies as a whole as to the cultural formulation, social negotiation, and institutional channeling of *ikigai,* and as to how they enable their members to sense the significance of their lives.

Ikigai in Three Societies: Societal Difference, Fate, and Cultural Formulation

In the following sections, I compare Japan, the United States, and Hong Kong in terms of the *ikigai* theory set forth above; but first, let me outline *ikigai* in these societies. Very broadly, Japan and the United States are in contrast in their *ikigai* formulations, with Hong Kong in the middle. The *ikigai* of men and women in the prime of life (twenty-five to sixty years old) whom we interviewed in all three societies tended to be work and family. However, the Japanese showed a marked gender division of *ikigai:* in Japan, the institutionally sanctioned values of men's commitment to company and women's commitment to family remain strong. In the United States and Hong Kong, there is less of a gender division: both men and women said they found *ikigai* in family as well as work. It seems expected that in both societies one proclaim that "my family is most important," but in actual daily life, this may not be the case, with work taking precedence (see Hochschild 1997).

Another important difference concerns religious belief. A significant minority of Americans and Hong Kongers found their *ikigai* in their Christian beliefs,[6] but few Japanese identified their ikigai with their religion (most often "new religions" such as Sōka Gakkai). Unlike Hong Kongers and Americans, Japanese thus (1) tended to show a more marked gender division in *ikigai,* and (2) tended not to find *ikigai* in religious belief. This may reflect the ongoing tendency in Japan to find one's deepest meaning within a defined role in one's primary this-world social group (see Lebra 1976, 67–90). In the United States, *ikigai* of work, family, and religious belief tended to be phrased in terms of "self-realization"; even if commitment to company or family was deeply valued, it was difficult to express this within the individualistic American vocabulary

(Bellah et al. 1985). In Japan, although a significant minority of those I interviewed spoke in individualistic terms as to what they lived for, the majority spoke in terms of commitment to company and family. In Hong Kong, those we interviewed often held a typically American way of thinking in their individualistic commitment to work, and a typically Japanese way of thinking in their group-oriented conception of family. In the pages that follow, I discuss these societies together in terms of our theory, rather than discussing them each in turn; but the reader should keep in mind these basic societal distinctions.

Let us turn to our theory, beginning with its initial phrase: "On the basis of culturally and personally shaped fate." One way in which culturally shaped fate is apparent in interviewees' words is as "that which is taken for granted": those cultural values that are seen as natural. In my interviews, the taken-for-granted was most apparent when it was transgressed. As an older American man said of the 1970s, "you marry, raise a family, go to the office every day, your wife stays home with the kids. ... That's what's you're supposed to do. ... When my wife said she wanted a divorce, it came as a total shock." His "common sense" had been overturned by the changing American cultural mores of that era. An older Japanese company employee assumed that his employment would continue until his retirement, but found, to his shock, that in the straitened economy of the late 1990s, such an assumption was no longer valid: he was laid off. "It wasn't supposed to be like this," he ruefully told me. Hong Kong "common sense" has also been changing, shaken by economic downturn in the early 2000s. In one college student's words, "It's shocking that even though I've gone to university, I might make less money than my father, who never went to secondary school." In all these cases, what was once taken for granted can be taken for granted no more, to the shock of those who must experience such a shift (and the shock of political upheaval and war can only be far greater). *Ikigai* is shaped within a taken-for-granted cultural world that might be subsequently transformed in later decades, shaking and perhaps shattering the very basis of one's *ikigai*.

"Individuals strategically formulate and interpret their *ikigai* from an array of cultural conceptions." While there are only a few *ikigai* generally held in the contemporary world—work, family, dream, religion, creative endeavor, country—there are a wide variety of cultural formulations of *ikigai*. One's *ikigai* of work, for example, can be justified in terms of the salary one earns, as is often the case in Hong Kong; in terms of the self-fulfillment that it may bring, as is often the case in the United States; or in terms of one's commitment to one's work group, as is often the case in Japan. These are stereotypes—all three justifications exist in all three societies—but do reflect dominant discourses within each of these societies.

For some people we interviewed, their formulations of *ikigai* come from beyond their own society—one may formulate and justify one's *ikigai* from an array of forms from the world over. I interviewed a Japanese executive who described her *ikigai* as found in her study of French existentialism ("On my deathbed, I want to be able to say that I've lived well.... No one will remember me a few years after I'm dead."). I interviewed an American Catholic nun who confided that she really felt closer to the Dalai Lama than to the Pope, and I interviewed a fifty-something Hong Kong Chinese rock musician who lived for the songs of Deep Purple. One extreme testament to the global "cultural supermarket" is John Walker Lindh, the Marin County teenager turned "American Taleban," a transformation apparently made possible through the internet (BBC 2002). A person in Japan, the United States, or Hong Kong can, indeed, potentially become anything or anyone in the world.

However, the dominant mass media in different societies emphasize a narrow range of messages—your American commuter is far more likely to be shaped by Rush Limbaugh than by Iranian mullahs, and the equivalent is true in Japan and Hong Kong. Theoretically, the availability of cultural formulations is huge, but in fact, one's society severely delimits their plausibility—people tend to be shaped by what media are most immediately available. This is not to say that media automatically reflect the dominant values of their society's social and institutional structures. In Japan, as we've discussed, mass media often discuss "living for yourself and not for your company" (Y. Yamada 1999), in terms echoed by some of those I interviewed, but companies continue to be structured as if the company is the ultimate locus of the individual's loyalty. In Hong Kong today, the dominant institutional voice is that of Hong Kong's loyalty to China; yet mass media such as *Apple Daily* poke fun at this view. In open societies, media offer multiple conflicting voices, which may help to shape *ikigai* in multiple, conflicting ways.

Ikigai in Three Societies: Social Negotiation, Institutional Channeling, Significance

"Negotiate these *ikigai* within their circles of immediate others." In all three societies, there is relativism in social relations. One cannot criticize others for their *ikigai:* "pursue whatever makes you happy" is a standard injunction. This attitude was strongest in the American context: several Americans I interviewed said, "It's my life. I can do what I want," a view hard to argue against in the United States, at least outside one's immediate intimates. In Hong Kong, relativism is also in play, except when it comes to family—paying a significant portion of one's salary to one's parents is not a matter of individual choice but of moral necessity for many young adults I know—but in other aspects of life, one is relatively free. In Japan, among some older people, relativism is rejected: there are certain ways in which one should live, involving sacrifice of "selfishness" for the sake of one's group, whether a man's work or a woman's family. But these assumptions are hotly contested by many other Japanese I interviewed, for whom personal freedom is most essential. Voices against *ikigai* relativism can be heard in the United States and Hong Kong as well—American evangelical Christians spoke of their disgust at the moral sinkhole into which they felt America had fallen, just as Hong Kong Chinese patriots spoke with disdain about their fellow Hong Kongers who feel no "love for the motherland"—but in Japan these voices seem most apparent. Nonetheless, *ikigai* relativism has more or less become the order of the day in all three societies—a relativism abetted by the fact that most people don't talk about what they live for to those they don't know well.

Within the more intimate world of one's immediate others, however, relativism is not generally adhered to. One of the most heated of these realms is that of gender roles. Negotiations of work and family responsibilities in the United States are frequent among couples. "There's a war that goes on between men and women," several American women I interviewed told me. In one's words, "men have never accepted that it's equally their responsibility to raise children, down to a nitty-gritty thing like, when a child needs something it will call its father as readily as it will call its mother, and Dad will respond." This woman's own divorce took place because her husband did not accept this responsibility (see Hochschild 1989).

In Japan, such negotiations have not occurred in more old-fashioned relationships ("my wife is like air to me," one older man said: essential for survival yet ignored) but are apparent in relationships among younger people. As one husband in his thirties told me, "Early in our marriage, my wife was always angry because I came home late from work. … She made me promise that … I'd have breakfast with the family no matter how late I came home the previous night." Hong Kong negotiations are similar, except that there is, in a middle-class context, a societal expectation of respect for wives; negotiations over the exact share of childcare and housework seem forestalled before this expectation of "chivalry." Even more important, there is the ready availability of foreign maids, which in effect frees middle-class wives to live for work, leaving the tedium of housework and childcare to hired help.[7] At the same time, the prevalence of "second wives" over the border in China for (typically) Hong Kong working-class men creates considerable gender tension; one young woman broke down in tears describing how, whenever her father is criticized by her mother, he runs off to be comforted by his mistress. I do not have space to further discuss the social negotiation of *ikigai* in these three societies, but this is an extraordinarily rich area for analysis.

"And pursue their *ikigai* as channeled by their society's institutional structures." One institutional structure is that of employment. In both the United States and Hong Kong, there is considerable employment mobility—people often change jobs and even careers. In Japan, for white-collar workers employed by large companies, lifetime employment remains the norm: the young person embarking on a career may have to assume that his choice will shape his entire life. This dominant institutional structure does not allow for flexibility of employment, with profound effects on the potential explorations of *ikigai* that young Japanese may undertake. Another example concerns gender. Aside from the fact that women's wages as compared to men's wages are lower in Japan than in Hong Kong or the United States, there is also the fact that Japanese tax laws discourage two spouses from working, by heavily taxing the second spouse's earnings beyond a certain minimum, thus "encouraging" married women to not work full-time (Mathews 2003, 216). Hong Kong immigration laws, on the other hand, allow for the employment of some three hundred thousand Filipina and Indonesian maids in Hong Kong, thus "encouraging" Hong Kong middle-class women to devote themselves to their careers (see Constable 1997). These institutional structures do not determine *ikigai*, since individuals who are sufficiently motivated and fortunate can overcome them. However, in large scale, they shape the *ikigai* of the members of any given society. For example, Japan's institutional structures favoring long-term employment for men and low compensation for women in the workplace powerfully encourage the maintenance of the de facto *ikigai* of "men living for work and women for family," despite the fact that a multiplicity of cultural voices in Japan argue against this.

"So as to attain and maintain a sense of the personal significance of their lives." The pursuit of significance is universal, but the forms that significance takes are matters of particular cultural shaping. I earlier mentioned three ways in which *ikigai* as work is formulated in the United States, Hong Kong, and Japan, in terms of self, money, and group, respectively; these reflect larger cultural shapings of significance in the three societies. Baumeister (1991, 365–70) has written of "the glorification of selfhood" in the American pursuit of life meanings: work and family have both been eroded, and so self becomes the bastion of value, with work and family justified only in that they fulfill the self. American *ikigai* justifications, Baumeister implies, are futile, despite the strength of American religious belief, in that the self cannot avoid death. In Hong Kong, gaining success in terms of money (Mathews and Lui 2001, 10), against a backdrop of familial loyalty, is the ultimate goal of many people's lives. Indeed, in a society of refugees, money and family are all that can be trusted. Hong Kong's civic values, of rule of law and governmental stability, can serve as no ultimate security, given an uncertain new world of linkage with China. In Japan, the ultimate valuation of one's group remains paramount, at least for some segments of the population; but even more than the two societies described above, Japan is in the throes of a "legitimation crisis" (in Habermas's 1973 term): in an age of economic downturn, the ideology of "surrendering self to group" has for many lost its meaning.

There are many alternative forms of the pursuit of significance in these societies; but these dominant forms reveal that all three societies suffer, in varying degrees, from a "legitimation crisis": the ties that bind individual to social order are frayed, their promise not fully believable. This may be a general contemporary malaise. Baumeister (1991, 360) coins the term "the mutual bluff" as describing the illusions set forth by self and society to maintain the self's illusion of a meaningful life. The frightening thing today is that so many people, in all three societies we have examined, know that these are illusions. And with this we may return to Max Weber's question asked earlier, of what binds self to society—a question for which today, more than ever, there seems to be no clear answer.

Conclusion: *Ikigai* as an Analytical Tool

I began this paper by discussing the existential basis of well-being, and offered *ikigai* as a way to get at this basis. Following a discussion of *ikigai* in Japan, I examined *ikigai* as a cross-cultural variable, and compared Japanese, Americans, and Hong Kongers as to the cultural formulation, social negotiation, and institutional channeling of *ikigai,* and the pursuit of significance via *ikigai.* Through such analysis, societies may be compared as to how they structure the pursuit of *ikigai.*

What can we conclude about *ikigai* and well-being in these three societies? The ranking of countries in the style of economists, public health experts, and psychologists seems a bit problematic for *ikigai.* No doubt *ikigai* may be more easily pursued in Japan, the United States, or Hong Kong than in Iraq or Somalia today, simply in that the former societies have a degree of affluence and security that the latter lack; but we cannot easily make finer gradations than this. Nonetheless, some general observations can be made. In Japan, institutions continue to demand a degree of suppression of the individual, even though the cultural discourse of individualism is widespread. Social pressure and institutional channeling may push young people towards following a set career path, and may push women towards living for family more than work. But while some Japanese are miserable at having made what they see as life-restricting choices (Mathews 1996, 82–87), and many young people are attempting to abandon the restrictive paths of their parents, other Japanese are happy being so cocooned, and having life laid out for them with few worries about "who they are" (Mathews 1996, 106–10).

In the United States, in contrast, a great degree of personal freedom is allowed in the pursuit of *ikigai;* for an unusual, talented person, this societal flexibility may enable them to fully develop their potential. However, while some Americans have used their freedom to change jobs and spouses to create happier lives for themselves (Mathews 1996, 87–92), others have suffered from too much freedom (Mathews 1996, 111–15); and one's own individual pursuit of freedom may leave a trail of others' emotional wreckage in its wake. In Hong Kong, there is an American-style freedom at work while at the same time a Japanese-style security in family.[8] Hong Kong has problems pertaining to *ikigai,* such as the high valuation given to money as a source of significance. There is also the fact that middle-class *ikigai* in Hong Kong is supported by the presence of maids from poorer societies, without which gender tension would no doubt be exacerbated. But Hong Kong does seem to allow career freedom on the basis of familial nurturance, in a sense a happy medium between the other two societies we have examined.

Different societies produce their own character types; selves are molded by their society, and recreate that society largely in accordance with that molding. These different character types may flourish in societies created after their own image. But there is a minority of people in each society who do not fit, who would be best suited to live in a society structured differently. Rather than ranking societies on a universal scale, the theory of *ikigai* explored in this chapter can enable us to glimpse the different relations of individuals to society within the sociocultural structurings of *ikigai.* If a broad range of individuals in any society can be profiled as to their *ikigai* using this structure, then a phenomenological profile of that society could emerge, and we could come to understand how different societies' cultural patternings, social relations, and institutional structures live within the minds of a diverse array of their members, structuring their pursuits of lives worth living. This would be valuable information that could make more subtle the comparison of societies worldwide as to well-being.

Notes

1. See, for example, Shostak (1981), Freeman (1979), and Crapanzano (1980), to mention three of a number of life histories that challenge but ultimately reward the efforts of the analyst seeking to understand the pursuit of significance in societies that substantially differ from those of contemporary global modernity.
2. This gap between language and experience is the case not just for anthropology, but for every discipline that investigates well-being. As compared to disciplines using questionnaires, anthropology, with its emphasis on interviews and participant-observation, goes further in the cross-cultural examination of well-being, but the gap between words and worlds necessarily remains.
3. This distinction between "self-realization" and "commitment to group" is interestingly played out in Dernè's chapter 6 and Jankowiak's chapter 7, with the former emphasizing "commitment to group" as a positive value and the latter "self-realization." These are, it seems, universals of human experience, with a given society's different values ranging between these poles of "self as a part of other selves" and "self as apart from other selves."
4. In Japan, unlike societies such as the United States or Australia, assuming career-track employment is generally possible only during a brief period of a few years during one's twenties. Thus, those who choose not to enter career-track employment may be making an irrevocable decision that will affect their entire lives (Mathews 2004).
5. I did all I could to minimize the possibility of overt dissembling, by talking with the people I interviewed for many hours over several meetings. But finally, if there was a contradiction between a person's beliefs ("Men and women are equal!") and behavior ("He gets angry when I don't cook his dinner!"), I could not address this unless I could interview both the person in question and his or her intimates. I did this wherever possible, but often I could not.
6. Most Americans are Christian, but many of the American Christians I interviewed did not see their religion as what was most important in their lives. On the other hand, only about 20 percent of Hong Kongers are Christian, but those who are Christian seem usually to make their religion the central focus of their lives.
7. There are many stories in Hong Kong of small children confusing their maids and their mothers, inconsolably crying "Mommy! Mommy! Come back!" when a maid's contract ends.

8. One indicator of this is divorce rates: Hong Kong's and Japan's divorce rates are both at 1.8 per thousand people, while the United States has the highest in the world, at 4.7 per thousand (*Economist* 2003).

References

BBC News. 2002. "Profile: John Walker Lindh." 24 January. http://news.bbc .co.uk/1/hi/world/americas/1779455.stm. Accessed 15 October 2003.

Baumeister, Roy. 1991. *Meanings of Life*. New York: Guilford Press.

Becker, Ernest. 1971. *The Birth and Death of Meaning: An Interdisciplinary Perspective on the Problem of Man*. 2nd ed. New York: Free Press.

———. 1974. *The Denial of Death*. New York: Free Press.

Bellah, Robert, et al. 1985. *Habits of the Heart: Individualism and Commitment in American Life*. Berkeley: University of California Press.

Constable, Nicole. 1997. *Maid to Order in Hong Kong: Stories of Filipina Workers*. Ithaca, NY: Cornell University Press.

Crapanzano, Vincent. 1980. *Tuhami: Portrait of a Moroccan*. Chicago: University of Chicago Press.

Durkheim, Emile. 1965 [1915]. *The Elementary Forms of the Religious Life*. New York: Free Press.

Economist, The. 2003. *Pocket World in Figures 2004*. London: Profile Books.

———. 2005. "A Survey of Japan." Oct. 8.

Freeman, James M. 1979. *Untouchable: An Indian Life History*. Stanford, CA: Stanford University Press.

Furiitaa kenkyūkai [Temporary workers' research group], ed. 2001. *Furiitaa ga wakaru hon!* [A book for understanding temporary workers]. Tokyo: Sūken shūppansha.

Habermas, Jurgen. 1973. *Legitimation Crisis*. Boston: Beacon Press.

Harris, Grace Gredys. 1989. "Concepts of Individual, Self, and Person in Description and Analysis." *American Anthropologist* 91 (3): 599–612.

Hochschild, Arlie Russell. 1997. *The Time Bind: When Work Becomes Home and Home Becomes Work*. New York: Metropolitan Books.

Hochschild, Arlie, with Anne Machung. 1989. *The Second Shift*. New York: Avon.

Iida, Fumihiko. 2004. *Ikigai no kyoshitsu* [Lessons on *ikigai*]. Tokyo: PHP kenkyūjo.

Kamiya, Mieko. 1980. *Ikigai ni tsuite* [About *ikigai*]. Tokyo: Misuzu shobō.

Kanamaru, Hiromi. 1999. *Jibun no tame no ikigai zukuri: nakama ga iru to konna ni chigau gojūdai kara no ikikata* [Creating ikigai for yourself: Life after fifty will be very different when you have friends]. Tokyo: Ichimansha.

Kobayashi, Tsukasa. 1989. *Ikigai to wa nanika? Jiko jitsugen e no michi* [What is ikigai? The path towards self-realization]. Tokyo: Nihon Hōsō Shuppan Kyōkai.

Lebra, Takie Sugiyama. 1976. *Japanese Patterns of Behavior*. Honolulu: University of Hawaii Press.

Marske, Charles E. 1987. "Durkheim's Cult of the Individual and the Moral Reconstitution of Society." *Sociological Theory* 5: 1–14.

Mathews, Gordon. 1996. *What Makes Life Worth Living? How Japanese and Americans Make Sense of Their Worlds.* Berkeley: University of California Press.

———. 2000. *Global Culture/Individual Identity: Searching for Home in the Cultural Supermarket.* London: Routledge.

———. 2003. "Can a 'Real Man' Live for His Family? *Ikigai* and Masculinity in Today's Japan." In *Men and Masculinities in Contemporary Japan: Dislocating the Salaryman Doxa,* ed. James E. Roberson and Nobue Suzuki, 109–25. London: RoutledgeCurzon.

———. 2004. "Seeking a Career, Finding a Job: How Young People Enter and Resist the Japanese World of Work." In *Japan's Changing Generations: Are Young People Creating a New Society?* ed. Gordon Mathews and Bruce White, 119–34. London: RoutledgeCurzon.

Mathews, Gordon and Tai-lok Lui. 2001. Introduction to *Consuming Hong Kong,* 1–22. Hong Kong: Hong Kong University Press.

Mita, Munesuke. 1984. *Gendai Nihon no seishin kōzō* [The spiritual structure of contemporary Japan]. Second edition. Tokyo: Kōbundō.

Mori, Shunta. 1999. "*Kankoku no kôreisha no ikigai*" [The *ikigai* of Korea's elderly]. In *Kôreisha no ikigai ni kan suru kokusai hikaku kenkyû* [Elderly *ikigai*: an international comparison]. Tokyo: Kōreisha noryoku kaihatsu kenkyūkai.

Nakano, Lynne and Moeko Wagatsuma. 2004. "Mothers and Their Unmarried Daughters: An Intimate Look at Generational Change." In *Japan's Changing Generations: Are Young People Creating a New Society?* ed. Gordon Mathews and Bruce White, 119–34. London: RoutledgeCurzon.

Niwano, Nikkyō. 1969. *Ningen no ikigai* [Human *ikigai*]. Tokyo: Kōsei Shuppansha.

Shiraishi, Eriko. 1998. *Seijinki shōgaisha no hattatsu to ikigai* [The development and *ikigai* of adults with disabilities]. Kyoto: Kamogawa Shuppan.

Shostak, Marjorie. 1981. *Nisa: The Life and Words of a !Kung Woman.* Cambridge, MA: Harvard University Press.

Takahashi, Yūetsu and Shūichi Wada, eds. 2001. *Ikigai no shakaigaku: kōrei shakai ni okeru kōfuku to wa nanika?* [The sociology of *ikigai*: What is happiness in an aging society?] Tokyo: Kōbundō.

Wada, Shūichi. 2001. "*Kindai shakai ni okeru jiko to ikigai*" [Self and *ikigai* in modern society]. In *Ikigai no shakaigaku: kōrei shakai ni okeru kōfuku to wa nanika?* [The sociology of *ikigai*: What is happiness in an aging society?] ed. Yūetsu Takahashi and Shūichi Wada, 25-52. Tokyo: Kōbundō.

Weber, Max. 1964 [1925]. "The Fundamental Concepts of Sociology." In *The Theory of Economic and Social Organization.* New York: The Free Press.

Yamada, Masahiro. 1999. *Parasaito shinguru no jidai* [The age of "parasite singles"]. Tokyo: Chikuma Shobō.

Yamada, Yūichi. 1999. *'Kaisha' yori mo 'jibun' ga katsu ikikata* [How to live so that you win out over your company]. Tokyo: KK besutoserā.

PART FOUR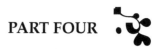

New Anthropological Directions

9

PLEASURE EXPERIENCED
Well-Being and the Japanese Bath
Scott Clark

> The heart asks pleasure first,
> And then excuse from pain.
>   Emily Dickinson

As physical beings, humans everywhere experience the world physically. Humans also have concepts of experiencing the world, and perhaps the universe, on other dimensions, spiritually and culturally and ranging from the climactic to the unnoticed. To achieve a sense of well-being, the experiences that are noticed need to be, on balance, positive. Pleasure is one positive experience, sensory pleasures among the most obvious. We notice when something feels good or pleasant, smells good, tastes good, sounds good, or looks appealing. Indeed, if we consider what well-being may mean, can we imagine it without sensory pleasures? In this chapter, I will look at a specific instance of sensual pleasure, the Japanese bath. This pleasure is physically sensed and, I will argue, much of the physical pleasure of that bath may be experienced by all humans, not just Japanese. But I will also show that the experience of the pleasure at the bath goes beyond the physical senses; embedded in Japanese culture, the act of bathing in the Japanese way by Japanese provides a broader sense of well-being as a Japanese person.

Pleasure, as I define it below, is positive, a component of happiness and, thus, well-being. Anthropology is particularly well positioned to study the relationship of pleasure and well-being. Disciplines including psychology, economics, business, and political science claim that well-being is fundamentally important, basing their claims on considerable data and recognizing that studying problems and their solutions alone is insufficient. Well-being is more than an absence of problems; it is a positive state that is pursued by humans. Anthropologists are well situated to contribute a cross-cultural perspective to these studies. I will show that methodology commonly used by anthropologists can enable us to gain a more fully developed understanding of pleasure as experienced by members of a society. Those understandings can be applied cross-culturally to understand well-being as a human experience. Indeed, if an anthropological-like approach is absent, human well-being is likely to be misunderstood.

I think pleasure is individualistic. "Japanese pleasure" does not exist.
(Conclusion of an interviewee, Summer 2003)

In my book on bathing (Clark 1994), I incidentally claimed that Japanese experience pleasure while bathing in a manner that is suffused with Japanese culture. Only after the book was published did I reflect on that claim and wonder what I meant by *pleasure*. Is pleasure individualistic and idiosyncratic, as the interviewee above concludes, or is it also cultural? Is the stimulation of the physical senses the basis of bathing pleasure, or is it something more? If there is a cultural component to pleasure, have anthropologists adequately addressed it? I am now somewhat further along the road to answering those questions than I was when they first occurred to me.

Intuitively, one suspects that there is a cultural component to pleasure. For example, one frequently hears reference to the pleasure of reading a good book, perhaps in front of a fire—the latter obviously sensual, but the former not so much. While not all individuals in a society may find pleasure in reading, certainly the society's culture must include, at a minimum, literacy and books for that particular pleasure to occur. It is safe to also claim that the fire in front of which one reads, especially in a walled room, would not be pleasurable in some climates. Therefore, components that make the experience pleasurable are at least partly derived from particular cultural and environmental contexts.

Before proceeding further, a definition of pleasure is necessary. Defining pleasure operationally has not proven easy. Definitions of pleasure that I have found seem to be based on an individualistically oriented perspective. Rozin critiques the *Oxford English Dictionary* definition ("condition of consciousness or sensation induced by the enjoyment or anticipation of what is felt or viewed as good or desirable") and adopts this one: a "positive experienced state that we seek and that we try to maintain or enhance," which, he argues, "stands for both a state of affairs and a dimension that they anchor" (1999, 111–12). This definition includes the experienced state and the seeking, maintaining, and enhancing of that state or dimension. Rozin's definition seems useful for my purposes, if we include within the "state of affairs," the settings, activities, and meanings—the cultural context—of seeking, maintaining, and/or enhancing a positive experienced state. It is the context that makes a cultural examination of pleasure possible.

Even simple examples demonstrate the importance of context. In June 2002, I had the *pleasure* of visiting several baths and saunas in Japan with friends. After soaking in a hot spring on one partly overcast day, our parked automobile was uncomfortably hot when we entered it. My impression was that the car's interior temperature was similar to the water temperature of the bath and certainly less than the temperature of the sauna located in a corner of the bathing area. After hearing expressions of discomfort from my friends and acknowledging a similar personal discomfort, I stated my impression of the relative temperature and asked my friends why the heat of the bath was pleasurable but the heat of the car was unpleasant. Various responses were given; one was trenchant: "Because it is a car" (*kuruma dakara*). In other words, our pleasure was very much dependent upon the context. Heat was an essential element of the pleasure that we sought and experienced in the bath; but heat alone was not sufficient to induce pleasure. The heat of the bath included the sensual feel of the water with its mix of naturally occurring minerals, the setting of the bath, the social nature of the experience, the symbolism of bathing at a hot spring, the recreation/leisure that we were seeking, etc. The heat of the car may have been pleasurable on a cold winter day, a different context. On this warm, early summer day, the heat was decidedly unpleasant, and we soon mitigated that by opening windows and turning on the air conditioner.

An initial search for insights into pleasure from anthropology has yielded little information. Standard references such as the Human Relations Area Files do not include pleasure as a category.[1] Some studies on emotion and culture refer briefly to pleasure. For example, Kitayama and Markus's (1994) edited volume on emotion and culture has two indexed entries to pleasure; several index entries exist for happiness and joy (also see Thin, chapter 1). This lack frankly surprised me. Perhaps it is just too common to engender study. Similarly, years ago, when I began a literature review about Japanese bathing, little existed beyond comments about its central importance in Japanese culture, with the exception of several studies of the history of bathing (see Clark 1994). Several professors at Japanese universities initially assisted me in trying to locate sources by Japanese academics. Each felt that someone must have done something fairly detailed, because they knew how important it was. But, we discovered almost nothing. David Plath, who studied enjoyment in "the after hours" in Japan, came across a sense by colleagues that such a study was trivial (Plath 1964), which may also be a partial explanation. Because anthropologists have not addressed pleasure directly, a good working definition for cross-cultural comparison does not exist.

Another difficulty that I have encountered with this examination of pleasure in Japan is finding an equivalent Japanese word. Sometimes when I am with Japanese who are experiencing something that I characterize as pleasure, they say *manzoku,* which is closer to "satisfying." Or other times, they may say *tanoshii* (akin to fun or enjoyment), *gokuraku* (paradise), *saikō* ("the best"), and *kimochi ga ii* (feels good). The latter is definitely associated with physical, sensual pleasure, while the first is more about a mental state. There exists a fairly formal word, *kairaku,* frequently used by academics and in translations of the word *pleasure* from English (perhaps other languages as well). But, I rarely heard *kairaku* used by Japanese speakers, unless we were self-consciously speaking about "pleasure" in a kind of stilted, formal sense. *Kairaku* apparently is a kind of specialized jargon developed to express a formalized concept of pleasure rather than a word commonly used to express pleasure as experienced. Perhaps if Japanese had a common equivalent to "pleasure" it would have been noticed and studied by at least foreign scholars, since its pursuit permeates so much of Japanese leisure time (and sometimes work).

Broadening my search to sociology and psychology yielded little more information that fits my purposes.[2] Both disciplines, like anthropology, have largely ignored pleasure, although psychologists have studied some of the physical manifestations related to the individual. Philosophy has a long tradition of discussing pleasure from at least as far back as Plato (Helm 2002; Perry 1967; Edwards 1979). But these tend to be theories about the universalism of pleasure. Philosophers, along with psychologists, argue or discuss aspects of the pleasure principle, the propensity to seek gratification of innate needs, and reducing pain—an individualistic orientation. Indeed, some philosophers and psychologists see the prospect of pleasure as the basis for all individual action. Turner (2000), in a review of psychology studies, argues that happiness, including pleasure, is a "primary" emotion. Other psychologists, anthropologists, and biologists have looked at pleasure as an environmental adaptation (Rozin 1999; Tiger 1992; Greenfield 2000). Commonly, however, pleasure is looked at as an individualistic, idiosyncratic, inner-mind phenomenon. Recently a number of psychologists have once again argued that psychology has too long ignored positive elements of the human psyche and must refocus on positive mental states, including pleasure; yet, the amount of research is still small (Seligman 1998; Maddux 2002; Kahnemann, Diener and Schwarz 1999; Rich 2001; Rozin 1999).

If pleasure is idiosyncratic, then anthropology will have little to contribute to the discussion. But consider the following account by Cathy Davidson, as she describes a pleasant ritual that takes place millions of times a day at hot springs, public baths, health centers, and private homes in Japan:

> The mood is quite happy, utterly relaxed.
>
> We sit naked on low wooden stools, soaping ourselves with the terry washcloths, rinsing with red buckets filled from the taps and poured over the body. The conversation is lulled, languid, like the water, like the steamy air.
>
> I finish washing my entire body and notice that most of the women from my group are still soaping a first arm. I slow down, going back again over my entire body, washing and washing, the soapy cloth, the warm water, the joking talking laughing atmosphere, the bodies. The women in my group are now washing a second arm. I slow down again, deciding I will try to do it right this time, Japanese-style, concentrating on a leg. I baby each toe, each toenail, each fold of flesh, noticing for the first time in years the small scar on the inside of my ankle, a muffler burn from a motorcycle when I was a teenager. I'm fascinated by this ritual attention to the body, so different from the brisk Western morning wake-up shower. When I finish (again) and go to shampoo my hair, I see that most of the women in my group are still scrubbing. I give up. It must take practice. I have never seen such luxuriant pampering of bodies. (Davidson 1993, 81–82)

At a Japanese hot spring, Davidson encounters bathing in a new way. Although she does not use the word *pleasure*, it is clear that the women are experiencing pleasure.

> "May I help you wash your hair?" Kazue-san asks, as I struggle to pour some water over my hair from the little red plastic bucket.
>
> "Please let me!" interjects one of the *obasan* ["auntie": older woman] who has been watching me for several minutes. She is very old, probably in her seventies or even eighties. ...
>
> [*Obasan*] squeezes shampoo into her hand and then rubs her palms together briskly. She's a pro. She massages the shampoo into my hair, the thick pads of her fingers making circles against my scalp. Then she lays one hand on my head, and starts clapping up and down on it with the other hand, making a sound like castanets as she works her hands over my head. It feels great. After about ten minutes, she chops with the sides of her hands over my head, my neck, and my shoulders, a kind of shiatsu massage.
>
> I think I could die at this moment with no regrets. I feel about four years old and totally at home, this tiny grandmother massaging my back and shoulders, my scalp and forehead. (Davidson 1993, 82–84)

Clearly, the hot spring experience is pleasurable to Davidson. She goes into the unusual (at least for a North American[3]) public bathing space and enjoys not only washing herself but also getting a shampoo from an elderly Japanese woman, a naked stranger. In the opening quotation, Davidson suggests a difference between the Japanese bath and the "Western" shower. The topic of bath pleasure allows us to examine the question of "Japanese pleasure." It is clear in the description above that a physical, sensual pleasure is being experienced. Davidson experiences at least part of the sensuality experienced by her expert companions. One wonders, however, if the "practice" Davidson humorously identifies includes learning a Japanese sense of pleasure.

My own first experience of Japanese bathing was at a public bath in the second half of the 1960s. At the time, the majority of Japanese did not have a bath at home and bathed in local bathhouses. These baths were located in virtually every urban neighborhood only a few minutes walk away from home. They were social as well as hygienic centers. By the mid-1970s, the majority of residences had their own bath, and the number of public bathhouses declined but remains abundant. Hot springs have always been popular places to bathe and in recent decades the numbers of those have increased tremendously because of drilling, to say nothing of baths at health centers, saunas, golf courses, ski resorts, and almost every other form of recreational area. Japanese bathe together as families and friends and co-workers; although the daily bath together with neighbors has declined, the opportunities to bathe with people other than neighbors has increased tremendously. Of course Japanese also bathe solo; the bath at home has become an important ritual-like act.

After my first pleasurable experience, I bathed whenever I could at public baths and hot springs. In the late 1980s, I conducted a yearlong study of bathing, interviewing people in my neighborhood about bathing and traveling around Japan talking with people of all ages and social strata in cities and rural communities. Soon after being introduced, whether professionally or socially, to Japanese people, the topic of my research is frequently mentioned by the person introducing me. Japanese are interested and frequently volunteer stories of their own bathing experiences, often inviting me to share with them a favorite bath. If we have time for an extended conversation, they frequently state that they have never talked so much about bathing, and almost inevitably add some comment about how much bathing has been a positive part of their lives. My decades-long experience bathing in Japan, incidental conversations about bathing, and systematic investigation using anthropological methods has deepened my understanding of bathing and the pleasure that Japanese experience.

In 2002, at an *onsen* (hot spring), I watched a Japanese man with his son, about three years old, share an hour of bathing. They were clearly enjoying each other's company as well as the sensual pleasures of bathing. At another *onsen*, I observed a man and his five or six-year-old daughter spend about forty minutes together at the bath. They were laughing and talking when they entered, seemed excited about getting to the bath, played in the tub, enjoyed washing, talked almost constantly, and exited the bath laughing, talking, and looking forward to getting back to the inn's room with *mama.*

At the time, I wondered if anyone socialized into dominant US culture would have the same pleasure at the *onsen* as these two men and their children. Was the pleasure exhibited "Japanese" or a general human pleasure? Most parents in the US do not bathe with their children beyond the infant stage. When relating instances such as those in the preceding paragraph, my American students are often surprised. Japanese expect to bathe with their children, indeed consider it an important part of a parent-child-family bonding. I have only been with two Americans who took their children to the bath with us. Both the American children and their parents were quite hesitant about bathing together. Although they enjoyed the experience, they did not seem to have an experience very close to those of the Japanese fathers and their children above. The experienced pleasure is situated within the larger context of the culture, the patterns of behavior, and the relationships and values of Japan.

From Davidson's essay we can well ask: Did she experience the same pleasure as the other women, some portion of it, or something else entirely? Is pleasure universal, cultural, idiosyncratic, or all three at once? Although my comparison of parents and children bathing may suggest that it is cultural, I argue that it is all three, but will focus primarily on the cultural.

The academic references cited previously make a strong case for the universality of pleasure. The arguments, however, are mostly based in neurological/physical theory. Indeed, both psychological research and common experience tell us that pleasures are in some sense personal and idiosyncratic. Conversely, the relatively larger literature on emotion and culture claims that emotions are culturally and socially contextualized (see Kitayama and Markus 1994). Psychologists (Segall et al. 1999) acknowledge the importance of the sociocultural context of pleasure. Pleasure, as defined earlier, has a social and cultural context where anthropology may make the largest contribution.

Japanese Pleasure

This is an initial attempt to identify elements that contribute to pleasure as experienced by Japanese, though some elements contribute to pleasure elsewhere. If pleasure is cultural (as well as individual and universal), then we should expect patterns roughly corresponding to cultural groups. Such an expectation is circular: culture delineates patterns of pleasure experienced culturally. The expectation, nevertheless, does lead to testable propositions, including: (1) pleasure and the culture in which it occurs will share many of the same features; and (2) while outsiders may experience some portions of culturally dependent pleasures, the degree to which they share the spectrum of pleasure with the insiders depends upon their familiarity with the culture.

That the second proposition is so seems obvious to me; it shares that quality with meaning and many other features of culture. In the Japanese *onsen*, Davidson experienced some pleasures with her companions—but not nearly all nor in the form that Japanese shared. In my work (1994), I outline my own emerging understandings of the bath, my changing perceptions of its meanings for Japanese, and my growing understanding of the pleasure of bathing for Japanese. In other words, I claim that my own "practice" with Japanese bathing has resulted in increasingly similar experiences to those of Japanese people. It is this participant-observation, the experience of bathing in Japan and understanding the cultural components of bathing, that make it possible for me to discuss their bathing pleasure. In general, anthropology's methods and practices can contribute to an understanding of pleasure cross-culturally.

Several features comprise a typical set for experiencing bathing pleasure for Japanese. Some features are obviously tied to bathing; others are common to Japanese pleasure in general. Once a more comprehensive view of Japanese pleasure emerges, it can be compared cross-culturally. This illustration of bathing and Japanese pleasure is not sufficient for that larger purpose, but I provide a framework to study Japanese pleasure, refine the concept, and broaden our understanding.

There are formalized Japanese bathing rituals such as *ubuyu* (baby's first bath), *yukan* (bathing after death), and religious purification rituals. Here, however, I will examine ritualistic, everyday bathing. This has the advantage of examining a daily activity for most Japanese, the disadvantage of infinite variation. Nevertheless, as with formal rituals, the daily ritualistic baths include common apparatus, regularized behaviors, and associated meanings, which allow analysis and explication beyond the individual to the society.

The context of pleasure is: *the settings, activities, and meanings of seeking, maintaining, and/or enhancing a positive experienced state.* The factors that emerge as important indicators of bathing pleasure are not isolated. They are part of the context and elements such as the "physical," and include the materials of the site, the equipment utilized, and bodily facets such as expressions, postures, feelings, and sensuousness. Each is somewhat affected by and affects the others; individuals are also affected by and affect other people—sometimes when they are not even present.

Bathing Paraphernalia

To begin, there are the "things" or equipment of the mundane bath necessary for a pleasurable experience:

- Basin—for holding water and for rinsing
- Bathroom—separate from the toilet, the bathtub is located here and includes space for washing outside of the tub; in some instances this bathing room or space is outdoors
- Bathtub—for soaking, equipped with means to supply large amounts of hot water through replacement or reheating
- Clean clothes—typically some sort of sleepwear or lightweight robe
- Dressing room—usually separated from the bathroom
- Mirror—located in the bathroom, an additional one is typical in the dressing room
- Shower—usually a showerhead on a flexible hose
- Soap and shampoo—advertising fully exploits the sense of physical pleasure related to these products
- Spigot—with running hot and cold water for filling the bathtub and basin
- Stool—for sitting while washing
- Time—usually each evening, from thirty minutes to an hour in duration, more frequent and longer at *onsen* or other bathing facilities
- Towel and washcloth—the latter longer than those in North America
- Water—hot and cold, in relatively copious amounts, water heating on-demand; a heater allows reheating of the water at will; in public baths hot water is constantly running and overflowing

The alphabetical order specifically suggests no priority of one over another. Of course, a bath could be completed without some items if necessary. The amount of water required for pleasure is relative to the situation; in a mountain campsite, even small amounts may be welcome, but at a public bath, huge amounts are expected. Other things such as brushes, razors, toothbrushes, sponges, etc. may be added, and usually are, on an individual basis.

An examination of this list shows only a few items not usually present in North American bathrooms: the separate dressing room, continually heated bathwater, basin, stool, and the amount of time. Each of these items may increase the pleasure of the bath regardless of whether one is Japanese or not. To exclude any of them reduces the pleasure of Japanese to an extent that tends to surprise my North American acquaintances. For example, even thirty minutes for bathing/showering seems somewhat extravagant to many of my friends in the US; but such a short bath seems like something less than proper to Japanese. Indeed they frequently refer to it disparagingly as a crow's bath (*karasu no gyosui*). Thus while not necessarily unique, the list is a minimal set expected by Japanese for a pleasurable bath, and the degree to which they are present or absent affects the level of pleasure.

The dressing room in a Japanese home is crowded with lavatory and laundry. Except in the smallest apartments (and hotel rooms), a toilet is not located in the bathing room. Washing is done outside the bathtub with a drain in the floor. A boiler maintains the heat of the bathwater. This contrasts with the constant cooling of North American bathtubs that require the addition of hot water from the tap. Having no conceptual limitation on the amount of hot water used is important (a relatively recent phenomenon) and significant for pleasure. Placing a limit on the amount of hot water would decrease the sense of luxuriousness that the bath offers. An old phrase, "use hot and cold water" (*yumizu no yō ni tsukau*), suggests plenty of everything—obviously associated with bathing, but the thought is extended to all luxury. The basin is plastic or, less commonly, wooden. It is useful as a receptacle in which to rinse the washcloth and pour water over the body—common before showerheads became available and frequently cited as one of the luxuries of public baths and hot springs. The stool allows one to sit comfortably while washing. The amount of time enhances the relaxation and pleasure of the experience. If the time, basin, stool, or heater is not available, expectations about the pleasure of the bath by Japanese will be decreased; the bath becomes something else, at least for Japanese—perhaps simply a sterile cleansing activity.

I have discussed each of the items in the list above in more detail in other places. This set of "things," along with individual items that can be added as desired, constitute the paraphernalia of a pleasurable bath. North Americans that I know who have taken a bath in a Japanese home also find them pleasurable. As a list of individual items, they do not tell us much about what may be "Japanese" about the experienced pleasure. As a group, they are important; individually, some of them can be eliminated on an occasional basis. I refer to them as a "typical minimum" because without them, the pleasure is reduced significantly. Thus, in the case of these things, they each contribute to the experience of pleasure; their absence significantly decreases the expected pleasure of bathing. Put another way, any single item is pleasurable in itself, but the set makes it a Japanese pattern for experiencing bathing pleasure. Non-Japanese may also find the set or portions of it pleasurable; but until they understand them as a set and how less or more of one or the other affects the overall balance, they may not be experiencing the pleasure in a way similar to Japanese.

I have used the word *things* here deliberately. It is easy to confuse this list with what I have labeled "the Setting." The Setting is a broader concept that can include companions, the materials, the season of the year, etc. Those all affect some aspects of the pleasure. These things are found in most contexts of bathing, whether alone or in groups, in summer or winter, and so on.

"Doing" the Bath

Bathing is more than simply using things. Japanese bathe. Bathing is an activity. Like the list of "things," there is a list of "doing." The following list is sequential:[4]

- Disrobe
- Rinse body thoroughly
- Soak in the bathtub until completely warm and perspiring profusely
- Scrub the body, beginning with the face working toward the feet
- Shampoo
- Prepare the bathing-room/space for the next bather
- Dress

Generally, this list does not look especially fruitful for understanding pleasure that is Japanese, as opposed to generalized pleasure. Even the sequence does not seem unusual. The only thing that stands out for a North American is that rinsing and washing the body take place outside the tub; the cleansing itself and the soaking in the hot water do not seem especially unexpected. A closer examination shows that perspiring followed by scrubbing may have significance, as indeed it does. The reader will also notice the order of washing the body and preparing the bathing-room for the next bather. I will examine these points further below.

Experiencing the Bath

As I suggest above, the context of bathing pleasure now becomes more complex. It is not so much the materials that are used or unique sensations that they produce in the body that makes Japanese pleasure. It is the combinations, the sets, the patterns together that combine in ways that have meanings for Japanese. For example, in the extended quote earlier, Davidson clearly enjoys the bath. Her clever statement, "It takes practice," is insightful as well as amusing. There is more to the Japanese pleasure of bathing than her personal expectations (and pleasure); experience counts.

Bathing, washing, and cleansing have numerous meanings embedded within them. In a previous study, I have shown that many of those meanings are associated with a sense of renewal (Clark 1994). Each of the following is renewed through bathing:

- Cleanliness/Purity
- Health/Vigor
- Identity as Japanese
- Life
- Relationships/Self/Status

Cleanliness is an obvious purpose of bathing; the feeling of being clean gives pleasure. The purification that is associated with water cleansing rituals (*misogi*) carries over into bathing. While the mundane practice of bathing is not thought of as sacred, Japanese do feel more than just physically clean after a bath. It is similar to removing shoes before entering the house. The practicality of keeping the home clean is obvious; protecting the home from pollution also underlies the practice. This becomes very clear when the circumstances are reversed: when a person fails to remove their shoes or take a bath, people react far more negatively than would be expected by a simple lack of cleanliness. The simple expression "dirty" (*kitanai*) is perhaps the most frequently heard, but it and others such as "disgusting" (*iya*) are accompanied by shudders and/or negative facial expressions that indicate a deeper feeling about missing a bath than when one says something like "my car is dirty." The feelings of cleanliness *and* purity contribute to inducing pleasure at the bath.

Health and bodily vigor are associated with bathing, which maintains and renews them. Perhaps the times when this is most apparent are when after an illness, the doctor informs the patient that they may begin bathing again. Both the proscription of bathing while ill and the marking of renewed health by its resumption show the association of bathing with good health. Last year a friend was finally told by her doctor that she could resume bathing after slightly more than three weeks (she did shower next to the bath for hygiene). Visiting with her the following morning, she told me that it felt so good to be clean again. She sighed contentedly and then stated that she finally felt well and that the bath really felt wonderful.

Perspiration is also frequently associated with health. Many advertisements, for example, use a perspiring face or body to indicate the good health associated with rigorous physical activity. Perspiration is thought to remove wastes and impurities from the body. Therefore, part of the pleasure of soaking in the hot water is to induce a sweat, which cleans the body internally. While wet underarms and a sweaty face at the office are not thought to be desirable or pleasurable, perspiring in the bath contributes to the concept of health and vigor and the pleasure of feeling that way, of well-being. My initial experiences at bathing brought many admonitions from people that I should get a good sweat up before I began to wash with soap, indicating that I would enjoy better health and enjoy the bathing more.

Many other things are associated with bathing and health. Casual perusal of popular magazines, medical journals, health columns in newspapers, etc., shows the close association of bathing, health, and pleasure.

Japanese today are very aware of the identification of their style of bathing as peculiarly Japanese. This was not always so. While regional variations in baths existed in premodern Japan, I have come across no evidence of an indigenous notion of a "Japanese" bath before the end of the feudal period. Many Japanese today, of course, assume an ancient bathing identity; but it appears to be a modern association. When Japan reopened to foreign interaction in the nineteenth century, one of the things that received attention (frequently negative) from foreigners was the public bath. When Japanese traveled elsewhere in the world, they missed their usual bath. A combination of these and other factors led to the association of their bathing style with their identity as Japanese. Both during my formal research of bathing and in countless informal discussions, Japanese claim bathing as a marker of their ethnic identity. Marking by itself may not give pleasure; however, their voluntary expressions of Japanese-ness associated with the pleasure of participating in a "Japanese bath" indicate that this has become an important aspect of bathing.

Customarily, life is marked by the first bath and funerary bath. In between, events may be marked by other baths, such as the one prepared in some parts of Japan by the household heir for his mother on her sixty-first birthday (*kanreki*). The Shinto purification rituals are also life affirming. Bathing rituals are not limited to the living, but in most cases are associated with the living or the connections to life. For example, in some areas, baths are prepared for returning ancestors at *obon;* the ancestors are visiting the living. These activities and beliefs form a context for the generalized, yet subtle and seldom-expressed association of bathing as an act of the living. I was somewhat surprised during my year of formal research on bathing at the number of people who, following an extended interview, said that apparently their life history was marked by the various baths they had enjoyed. To be sure, some of the bathing stories related to me were not about enjoyable conditions, such as those taken under extreme conditions in combat or after the fire-bombing of cities. They recalled those baths in the context of an enjoyable, pleasurable event during a difficult time.

Everyone in Japan is aware of the traditional rule that sex and age order is followed for bathing. Not everyone is aware that this rule was rarely followed (Clark 1994). The presence of the rule, however, signals that social relationships are associated with bathing and reflects status relationships in the household. Bathing with children and grandchildren, bathing the elderly, preparing the bath, and leaving the bath in a state that is pleasurable to others are all part of domestic relationships associated with the bath. These activities are sometimes onerous, but most times pleasurable. Certainly many people have fond memories and experiences of bathing together at home. Even when people bathe alone at home, they are often keenly aware of the relationships that they must maintain with others and demonstrate them by the way that they prepare the bath for the next person before they exit the bathroom.

Even though travel, hiking, a golf outing, a ski trip, etc. frequently includes a bath with friends, except when children are small, bathing in Japan today is most commonly an individual activity. As such, the pleasure is most commonly an individually enjoyed pleasure that renews the sense of self and of well-being. A person bathing alone luxuriates in the pleasures as an individual (even at a public bath when they come alone). A growing body of literature in psychology emphasizes the collective versus individual orientation as a major factor in cross-cultural differences of well-being (Lopez et al. 2002; Diener and Suh 1999; Markus and Kitayama 1991; Suh 2000; Kitayama and Markus 2000), a trend that stems from an interesting cross-cultural study (Hofstede 1980). In his study of IBM employees around the world, Hofstede proposed a dimension (among others) of individualism—collectivism for comparison,[5] a dimension singled out for special emphasis in a number of subsequent studies.

Suh (2000) collapses East Asians into a group and asserts that they are less happy than North Americans. Happiness is, of course, different than pleasure; but pleasure contributes to happiness. Suh asserts that the difference is due to the relatively more individualistic orientation of North Americans. In the same volume, Kitayama and Markus state "Japanese may be primed relatively more to an arousal dimension than to a pleasantness dimension when experiencing emotions" (2000, 139). The arousal dimension refers to the positive and negative emotions aroused in others that then affect their own sense of well-being. They argue that Japanese, therefore, strive to keep positive and negative emotions in a balance. These three authors are examining the broad concept of well-being rather than the narrower one of pleasure. A general impression that derives from their research and the research that they review is that Japanese may experience less pleasure than North Americans. The authors *do not* state it that way nor do I think that they intend to leave that impression; certainly the impression is not correct. My use of the bath as an example of pleasure shows that Japanese in fact actively pursue pleasure, individually *and* collectively. The point I want to emphasize is that a cross-cultural comparison of pleasure is not sufficient on an individualist-collectivist dimension alone. Japanese enjoy baths individually *and* in social groups. Anthropology can contribute to the understanding of well-being that may be glossed over by the cross-cultural methods most commonly employed by psychology and other disciplines. It is not so much that the conclusions cited above are wrong, as that they are far from complete and can lead to mistaken inferences.

Social bathing is extensive in Japan today, whether it is a company outing or two friends after dinner. Bathing together signals a close relationship and building a closer relationship. Social differences are thought to be minimized at a bath. Social bathing is nearly always said to be pleasurable.

I have thus far noted much of the context of the Japanese experience of pleasure while bathing. I have suggested that the Settings, Activities, and Meanings provide the cultural context of pleasure. Figure 9.1 is meant to suggest that these are intertwined aspects of pleasure and cannot be separated; aspects can be identified for heuristic purposes, but all are parts of a whole. I have also mentioned in the narrative

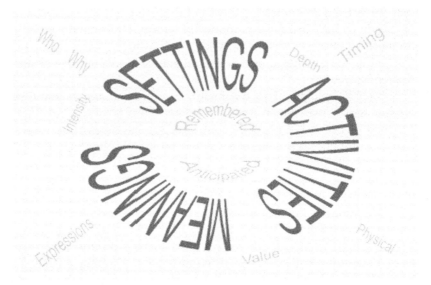

Figure 9.1 The Context of Pleasure

above some of the observations that help us to understand the extent of pleasure and its components.

A summary of the key points of the pleasure of bathing for Japanese are in Table 9.1. The table by itself does not explain why each element is important or the way that it is important.

I have used this framework in my analysis and it shows those aspects that I have found to be important. But it barely indicates pleasure as an experience. As should be readily apparent, Japanese pursue the experience of pleasure actively and regularly. The most common expressions of the activity are, not surprisingly, about the physical, sensual pleasures of the bath: the feeling of a cold autumn wind on bare skin and the tingle as one slithers into the hot water, the smooth slipperiness or caustic properties of mineral baths, the steam evaporating from flushed skin, the scents of soaps and minerals, the touch of a hand on the shoulder as one's companion braces to vigorously scrub your back, the pleasant sting of a thorough scrubbing, the balance of a young child on one's knee while telling stories in the tub, the sounds of water. . . . Sensuality is an important component of bathing pleasure, and there are many terms and phrases used repeatedly to describe these experiences.

An important point of these expressions and descriptions of pleasurable moments is that Japanese seek physical pleasure and indulge in it. That most Japanese seek such indulgent pleasure *every* day is not considered excessive or abnormal. The pursuit of this pleasure is seen

Table 9.1 Elements of Pleasure

CONTEXT			Evaluative Markers[5]
SETTING	ACTIVITIES	MEANINGS	
Basin	Disrobe	Cleanliness/	Time: when, how
Bathroom	Rinse	Purity	often, how long,
Bathtub	Soak	Health/Vigor	seasonal, etc.
Clothing	Scrub	Identity	Who: alone, with
Companions	Shampoo	Life course	whom
Dressing room	Tidy up	Relationships	Where: home,
Location	Dress	Self	resort, hotel,
Mirror	*Bathe with others*	Status	outdoors, etc.
Nature/Season	*Relax*		Body Expressions:
Shower	*Reminisce*		facial, pose,
Soap and	*Plan*		touch, etc.
shampoo			Linguistic &
Spigot			extra-linguistic
Stool			expressions
Time			Self reports: depth,
Towel &			value, intensity
washcloth			Remembered: why
Water (hot and			it is remembered
cold)			Anticipated: what
			is anticipated

as essential to well-being; the meanings associated with bathing are, indeed, fundamental components of well-being.

To relate a brief example of this pursuit of experiencing pleasure, in 1994 I was invited to accompany three women friends on an outing to Takayama, an old castle town in the high mountains. We left after work and headed toward a hot spring deep in the mountains. One woman brought along a plethora of treats and drinks to consume in the car. Another prepared a purse to which we all contributed a sum of money to cover common expenses such as a room, meals, and gas. A third woman drove. On the way we stopped at a noodle shop that had recently been featured in a television show, and then at a well-known mountain view. These caused us to arrive at the inn at a late hour. We ate and then bathed in both indoor and outdoor baths (with wonderful stones, wood, architecture, and views) and then talked and laughed late into the night, and then went to bathe again. *"Ii yu da na," "hada ga sube sube," "kimochi ga ii," "sukkiri shita," "tsukare ga torimashita," "saikō," "kirei," "suteki,"* —"the water is great," "my skin is smooth," "it feels good," "I am refreshed," "my tiredness is gone," "it does not get any better that this," "beautiful view," "wonderful" — and other expressions poured through the conversation along with sighs, stretches, and other signs of contentment and enjoyment. Morning found us bathing again, eating breakfast, lingering over coffee, and once again on the road to Takayama. We shopped in their favorite shops and enjoyed dining at a well-known restaurant. By late afternoon, I was exhausted and noted that the others seemed tired. But it had been a thoroughly enjoyable day. We hopped in the car and started on the journey home. About an hour from home, we stopped again at a hot spring for a refreshing soak in the waters. Once again, words and other expressions indicating pleasure came spontaneously. These women planned this trip and invited me along since I happened to be in the area at the time and they knew from past experience that I would enjoy going. The stay at the hot spring inn was quite expensive, more so than the amounts that they spent on shopping. The time away from families was partly relief from responsibility, but also meant that chores were piling up while they were away. They were pursuing pleasure/enjoyment and expressed pleasure in a number of ways the entire trip, and again the next few times that we corresponded or saw each other. These three women are close friends, and the primary reason expressed for their rather frequent trips is *tanoshimanakya*, "We have to have fun," implying that it is necessary for a good life, for well-being.

The importance of the sensual aspects of the pleasure probably cannot be overemphasized; however, to neglect or ignore the broader meanings and situations that provide pleasure in more than physically sensual ways distorts an understanding of the pleasure experienced by *Japanese bathing* (to say "the Japanese bath" here would separate the physical and/or social setting too far from the total context of the activity by Japanese). Indeed, stripped of the context, I suspect that Japanese may find the physical sensuality excessive and unpleasant; however, since that separation is not actually possible, my suspicions and the occasional expressed opinions to that effect that I have heard from Japanese are speculative.

Bathing Pleasure, Other Pleasures, and Well-Being

I have made a case that the pleasure experienced by Japanese while bathing is culturally situated. One needs to be situated in that culture in order to experience it as a Japanese person does. Davidson is an example of an outsider who experienced great pleasure at the Japanese bath, but while she shares some of the pleasure, especially the physical pleasure that her Japanese companions do, she did not possess enough of the cultural context to experience it all. Still, the example shows three aspects of pleasure: some pleasure may be experienced because of physical stimulations, some pleasure requires a cultural context to experience, and individual experience influences pleasure.

The first of the above (experience of pleasure is a human trait) is well established and the latter is obvious (no one but Davidson would have the experience to remember the events that led to the scar on her leg and whether to interpret the memory as pleasurable or not). Just as obviously, much of what makes Japanese bathing pleasurable is closely tied to the activity itself. Much more research will be required to see if a list of some elemental factors may be identified that are common to all, or at least most, pleasures experienced by members of Japanese culture. I suspect that the list will look somewhat similar to a description of Japanese culture itself; in other words, it will reflect Japanese culture and will have features that perhaps are not unique to Japan but, as a pattern, are a set that is identifiable as Japanese.[7]

There is a large popular literature describing various pleasures in Japan. My somewhat limited research into academic resources suggests that the topics are similar to those available in English, i.e., the physical/psychological aspects of pleasure, with much less about the social/cultural context (for example, Hironaka 2003).

Pleasure is a universal human experience; it is experienced individually and socially, and is a component of a sense of happiness and the broader state of well-being. Some aspects of pleasure are individual, but much pleasure is culturally shaped and informed. Here, I have identified aspects of a commonly experienced pleasure in Japan and show how that pleasure is culturally situated—how the settings, activities, and meanings are important to experiencing it as Japanese and understanding it as an anthropologist. I have also shown that some aspects of the pleasure may be experienced by an outsider without this specific knowledge, but have argued that the pleasure experienced by the typical outsider is somewhat distantly removed from that of the cultural members. I do not argue that an outsider cannot become an insider or that the outsider cannot learn to experience pleasure within the range of insiders' experience. Actually, I have shown the opposite: using the techniques and methodology of anthropology, we can understand pleasure in "other" societies and then compare them cross-culturally, contributing to an understanding of well-being.

Notes

1. A keyword search of the eHRAF, http://www.yale.edu/hraf/, showed 2311 matches in 719 documents and includes such phrases as, "It is a pleasure to meet you." A narrowed search using the "pleas*" with wildcard and the OCM code "152" (Drives and Emotions) showed only 135 matches in 75 documents. This is a very small showing considering the size of the database. A search of the Anthropological Index Online, http://aio.anthropology .org.uk/cgi-bin/uncgi/search_bib_ai/anthind, showed 39 matches. The bulk of the references are similar in nature to the HRAF, or more specifically to sexual pleasure.
2. I wish to particularly thank John M. Robson, Library Director, John A. Logan Library, Rose-Hulman Institute of Technology, for his generous help in locating sources.
3. I explicitly make comparisons to North America and the United States not because it is a standard, but because it is where I live and work.
4. Most instructions for bathing in Japan state that one should wash before entering the bathtub. The word for "wash" (*arau*) is used interchangeably with what would be a closer gloss, "rinse." In my observations and interviews, unless grime is visible on the body, the most frequent order is soaking first. The important feature is to be ritually (if not medically) "clean." In either case, a similar pleasure may be induced.
5. On this dimension, Hofstede placed the Japanese at about the middle point among the 66 countries studied. The US was the extreme point on the individualistic side.
6. I have included a column labeled Evaluative Markers for evaluating data. See Guichard-Anguis (2002) for a detailed analysis of changing motivations for visits to two *onsen* over time.
7. In some ways this is similar to Cox's (2002) analysis of "Is there a Japanese way of playing?"

References

Clark, Scott. 1994. *Japan, A View from the Bath*. Honolulu: University of Hawaii Press.

Cox, Rupert. 2002. "Is There a Japanese Way of Playing?" In *Japan at Play: The Ludic and the Logic of Power*, ed. Joy Hendry and Massimo Raveri, 169–85. London: Routledge.

Davidson, Cathy N. 1993. *36 Views of Mount Fuji: On Finding Myself in Japan*. New York: EP Dutton.

Diener, Ed and Eunkook M. Suh. 1999. "National Differences in Subjective Well-Being." In *Well-Being: The Foundations of Hedonic Psychology*, ed. Daniel Kahneman, Ed Diener, and Norbert Schwarz, 434–50. New York: Russell Sage Foundation.

Edwards, Rem B. 1979. *Pleasures and Pains: A Theory of Qualitative Hedonism*. Ithaca, NY: Cornell University Press.

Greenfield, Susan. 2000. *The Private Life of the Brain: Emotions, Consciousness, and the Secret of the Self.* New York: John Wiley & Sons.

Guichard-Anguis, Sylvie. 2002. "From Curing and Playing, to Leisure: Two Japanese Hot Springs: Arima and Kinosaki *Onsen.*" In *Japan at Play: The Ludic and the Logic of Power,* ed. Joy Hendry and Massimo Raveri, 245–58. London: Routledge.

Helm, Bennett. 2002. "Felt Evaluations: A Theory of Pleasure and Pain." *American Philosophical Quarterly* 39 (1): 13–30.

Hironaka, Naoyuki. 2003. 快楽の脳科学： いい気持ち」はどこから生まれるか．NHKブックス，東京：日本放送出版協会，8月，976 [*Pleasure and Science of the Brain: "Feeling Good," Where Does It Come From?*] Tokyo: Japan Broadcasting Publication Association / NHK Books, August.

Hofstede, Geert. 1980. *Culture's Consequences: International Differences in Work-Related Values.* Newbury Park, CA: Sage Publications.

Kahneman, Daniel, Ed Diener, and Norbert Schwarz, eds. 1999. Preface to *Well-Being: The Foundations of Hedonic Psychology,* ix–xii. New York: Russell Sage Foundation.

Kitayama, Shinobu and Hazel Rose Markus, eds. 1994. *Emotion and Culture: Empirical Studies of Mutual Influence.* Washington, DC: American Psychological Association.

Kitayama, Shinobu and Hazel Rose Markus. 2000. "The Pursuit of Happiness and the Realization of Sympathy: Cultural Patterns of Self, Social Relations, and Well-being." In *Culture and Subjective Well-being,* ed. Ed Diener and Eunkook M. Suh, 63–86. Cambridge, MA: MIT Press.

Lopez, Shane J., Ellie C. Prosser, Lisa M. Edwards, Jeana L. Magyar-Moe, Jason E. Nuefeld, and Heather N. Rasmussen. 2002. "Putting Positive Psychology in a Multicultural Context." In *Handbook of Positive Psychology,* ed. C.R. Snyder and Shane J. Lopez, 700–14. New York: Oxford University Press.

Maddux, James E. 2002. "Stopping the 'Madness': Positive Psychology and the Deconstruction of the Illness Ideology and the *DSM.*" In *Handbook of Positive Psychology,* ed. C.R. Snyder and Shane J. Lopez. New York: Oxford University Press.

Markus, Hazel Rose and Shinobu Kitayama. 1991. "Culture and the Self: Implications for Cognition, Emotion, and Motivation." *Psychological Review* 98: 224–53.

Perry, David L. 1967. *The Concept of Pleasure.* Hague: Mouton & Co.

Plath, David W. 1964. *After Hours: Modern Japan and the Search for Enjoyment.* Berkeley and Los Angeles: University of California Press.

Rich, Grant Jewell. 2001. "Positive Psychology: An Introduction." *The Journal of Humanistic Psychology* 41 (1): 8–12.

Rozin, Paul. 1999. "Preadaptation and the Puzzles and Properties of Pleasure." In *Well-Being: The Foundations of Hedonic Psychology,* ed. Daniel Kahneman, Ed Diener, and Norbert Schwarz, 109–33. New York: Russell Sage Foundation.

Segall, Marshall H., Pierre R. Dasen, John W. Berry, and Ype H. Poortinga. 1999. *Human Behavior in Global Perspective: An Introduction to Cross-Cultural Psychology.* 2nd ed. Needham Heights, MD: Allyn & Bacon.

Seligman, Martin E.P. 1998. "Building Human Strength: Psychology's Forgotten Mission." *The APA Monitor* 29 (2).

210 • *Scott Clark*

Suh, Eunkook M. 2000. "Self, the Hyphen between Culture and Subjective Well-being," In *Culture and Subjective Well-being*, ed. Ed Diener and Eunkook M. Suh, 63–86. Cambridge, MA: MIT Press.
Tiger, Lionel. 1992. *The Pursuit of Pleasure*. Boston: Little, Brown & Company.
Turner, Jonathan H. 2000. *On the Origins of Human Emotions: A Sociological Inquiry into the Evolution of Human Affect*. Stanford, CA: Stanford University Press.

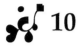 10

SELFSCAPES OF WELL-BEING
IN A RURAL INDONESIAN VILLAGE

Douglas Hollan

Many would agree that the state of being well has certain biological and social correlates. It is hard to be well if one is starving, if one is in chronic pain, or if one is the victim of assault or lives in constant fear of assault. But people who are not starving, who are not in chronic pain, and who do not live in fear of assault can tell us how miserable they are. So whatever well-being is (see introduction to this volume), it entails more than the fulfillment of basic biological and social needs.

In this chapter I argue that at the individual level, being well is inherently a contingent, subjective state that varies through space and time. To admit that well-being is subjective does not mean that it cannot be studied using traditional methods of participant observation and interviewing, nor to deny the prospects for comparative analysis. But it does demand that our investigations take a person-centered perspective (see Levy and Hollan 1998; Hollan 2000, 2001); that is, that they attempt to understand how the world is felt and experienced from the subject's point of view. I begin by explaining why well-being is so subjective and contingent, and introduce the concept of a "selfscape." I then present the idea that despite this contingency, all societies establish gradients of well-being in which certain kinds of routines or activities are given positive valence and encouraged while others are given negative valence and discouraged. In the following two sections, I analyze the contingency and variability of well-being in a rural Toraja community in the mountains of South Sulawesi, Indonesia. I conclude by summarizing the argument and offering suggestions for future research.

Why Well-Being is Subjective

Well-being is subjective and contingent because, in my view, it is related to the evolution of a human self-system that is constantly evaluating its condition, for survival purposes, relative to its own body, to other people, and to the world. All humans possess this basic biological ability to evaluate and monitor themselves (Hallowell 1955), but because self-systems only emerge and develop in interaction with particular social and physical worlds, they will differ from one another in both predictable and idiosyncratic ways.

In *Descartes' Error* (1994) and in *The Feeling of What Happens* (1999), the neuroscientist Antonio Damasio reminds us just how deeply the mind is rooted in the body and its biological processes. He emphasizes how dependent the mind and survival are upon continuously updated representations of the body and its relative health or illness, and how these representations "qualify" our perceptions of the world. For example, sick or hungry people are likely to act differently, to engage the environment differently, and to experience and perceive the behaviors and intentions of others differently than those who are healthy and satiated. In the later chapters of the first book and throughout the second, Damasio begins to speculate about the origins and maintenance of the self and consciousness. He suggests that neural representations of the self must be continuously updated and modified in a manner similar to that of bodily processes, and speculates that the earliest representations of the self very likely emerge from, or coincide with, representations of the body as it interacts with the world. Thus neural representations of the body, self, and world are inextricably tied together through complex emotional states and processes, all of which must be continuously updated and modified as they stimulate and impinge upon one another. The brain creates the phenomenological *illusion* of an ongoing, unified self as it represents fluctuating body and emotional states in interaction with a constantly changing environment, but it really is only an illusion, since the self-system itself, and its sensing of pleasure and pain, wellness and unwellness, is never static but is always dynamically related to the changing states of body and world it monitors.

Thus the self-system, and by implication one's awareness of one's own state of wellness or unwellness, is a dynamic and ever-changing product of the interaction of body/brain and experience. Without a body/brain, there is no experience. Without experience, without engagement in the culturally constituted and variable world, there is no emergence of self-processes, and consequently, no awareness of wellness or lack of wellness (Hollan 2004).

Implications for the Study of Well-Being

There are important implications in all of this for the study of well-being. One is that well-being must be highly contingent, depending on how the self-system is mapping itself at any given moment relative to changing states of body and environment and the interactions between the two. This mapping process is complex. In part, it is constrained by biological "values" of the body that have evolved in our species over an extended period of time, such as sensitivity to particular kinds of pleasures and pains and the physiological limits of cellular homeostasis (see Hinton 1999). As Damasio has suggested, the brain's moment-to-moment mapping of the body's internal dynamics is itself a hugely complicated process. But the body does not exist in a physical, social, or cultural vacuum. Indeed, the self-system maps the body as it moves through a culturally constituted world, which, like the internal dynamics of the body, is characterized by dynamic states of both stasis and change and is sensed and perceived through a cultural lens. Moreover, the culture through which the self-system senses and evaluates itself is not uniformly given, but is distributed across the social landscape (see Schwartz 1978) and is internalized to varying degrees by any given person. For example, as we shall see in a later section, not all Toraja internalize the belief in supernatural retribution to the same degree, and those who do, do not always embody or enact the belief in the same way.

But the complexities do not end here. As the self-system maps and evaluates the body as it moves through the culturally constituted landscape, it simultaneously maps a memoryscape of the body and self interacting with the world. Some of this mapping is conscious. A person thinks, "these artifacts or activities or people are familiar or unfamiliar; they have made me happy or unhappy or healthy or sick in the past." But much of it is nonconscious or unconscious. Psychoanalysis and the cognitive and neurosciences have taught us that consciousness captures but a small part of what the self and body/brain "know" about people and objects in the world. Implicitly and nonconsciously, we are always relating or associating these current experiences to our representations and constructions of past experiences.

Sometimes these associations are relatively direct and straightforward: without being consciously aware, we avoid or act aggressively towards artifacts or activities or people who have made us sick or unhappy in the past; we approach or actively embrace those that have made us happy or healthy. But other times, our nonconscious associations to the culturally constituted landscape are more convoluted and obscure, as psychoanalysis suggests. Without conscious awareness, people may attempt to dominate or control or even embrace those artifacts or activities or people that have frightened or hurt them in the past, in a compensatory way. For example, someone may become a soldier or police officer or football player to compensate for an inner sense of weakness or vulnerability. On the other hand, people may flee or avoid or ignore artifacts or activities or people that pose no "objective" threat to them because they have nonconsciously and erroneously associated them to actual or imagined experiences of the past that *have* posed some threat. For example, a person may be prone to criticize or avoid present-day authority figures, regardless of their actual behavior, because of negative experiences with such authority figures in the past. As Freud suggested, the self-system can become divided against itself, and its interactions with the world characterized by emotional states of ambivalence and conflict.

Thus the self-system is constantly mapping its own representations of its own past experiences onto the space and time of the contemporary culturally constituted world. I refer to these moment-by-moment mappings as *selfscapes*. The complexity and contingency of selfscapes pose daunting analytical challenges for the study of well-being. Because they develop in worlds that are saturated with multiple and conflicting values, they themselves are inevitably value-laden; people can only be well or unwell relative to some set of internalized values. Because they occur through time and across culturally constituted space, they themselves may conflict and contradict one another: for example, what promotes happiness and well-being at one moment, in one context, at one stage of life may not do so at another moment, in another context, at another stage of life. And because self-systems grow and develop epigenetically—that is, because their earlier experiences partially shape the way they respond to later experiences—people's selfscapes must differ from one another even in relatively small, monocultural communities, since people's life experiences will vary along dimensions of age, gender, status, birth order, idiosyncratic experience, and so on.

From this perspective, being well has a lot to do with the relative "fit" between a person's mind/body and the physical and social world. It is hard to be well if one's basic biological needs are not being satisfied, but one can be equally "unwell" if one is alienated from one's family or community or too often experiences humiliation, shame, fear, or anxiety—even if one is otherwise biologically fit. It is important to note that the poorness of fit between people and their social worlds can come about for several reasons. One can be excluded from the activities or routines that one finds most appealing or meaningful. One may exclude oneself from such appealing activities and routines, due to excessive shyness, shame, or inner conflict. Or, the activities or routines one *has* become embedded in are experienced as painful, unpleasant, or unfulfilling. Either lack of involvement or overinvolvement in the social world can become a problem for people.

Social and Cultural Gradients of Well-Being

While individual selfscapes are variable and contingent, in all communities they unfold in worlds that are socially and culturally organized in particular ways—no matter how swiftly these patterns of organized life might be changing as a result of larger-scale political and economic forces. Intentionally or not, all communities establish zones or gradients of well-being in which certain kinds of routines or activities are given positive valence and encouraged, while others are given negative valence and discouraged. Of course from the individual's point of view, the valence of some activities is mixed. Communities attempt to reward participation in some activities or routines, thought to benefit the individual or group over the long term, even though they may bring some short-term frustration or pain from the individual's point of view. Schools and other forms of formal education are good examples of activities that evoke ambivalent reactions from people in many parts of the world. Some activities or routines acquire a negative valence not because they are actively discouraged, but simply because they are not positively valued or encouraged. For example, teaching in the US is not actively disparaged per se, but because its prestige is not as high as many other professions, many people will avoid it or prefer to work in some other way.

Thus all communities create zones of activities and engagements for people that affect their sense of well-being in relatively positive or negative ways. As people move through the course of a day and traverse the socialscapes around them, as they move from one location to another and engage with various types of people and activities, they feel more or less safe and secure, more or less stimulated and engaged, more or less well or unwell. Almost all communities attempt to establish some form of "safe haven" for people—areas or activities in which people's basic social and emotional needs are fulfilled and in which they are protected from too much stress and anxiety. Households and family and friendship groups often serve this function. Conversely, there are zones or activities in all communities in which livelihoods and reputations are at stake, in which egos, if not bodies, can get bloodied and bruised, such as in the very public, and often contentious, division of sacrificial meat at a Toraja funeral. The contours of these socialscapes and the rules for navigating them will vary from culture to culture. Although individuals may, and often do, respond to these zones in different ways (as I suggest in a later section), the zones themselves have a certain stability for the simple reason that many of them are institutionalized through custom or law and so persist beyond the lifespan of individuals.

Gradients of Well-Being in a Toraja Village

Despite rapid growth and change in the market towns of Rantepao and Makele, rural Toraja hamlets in highland Sulawesi, Indonesia remain scattered among steeply terraced rice fields and patches of forest and gardens, much as they did when I conducted extended field work there in the 1980s (see Hollan and Wellenkamp 1994, 1996). As one walks through these mountains or drives along one of the handful of rough, unpaved roads that slice through them, one sees that hamlets consisting of two or three to up to a dozen households, most without running water or electricity, are strategically placed to accommodate the back-breaking cultivation of rice. Such cultivation remains the primary means of livelihood for those who have stayed in the countryside and have been unwilling or unable to migrate to city and town.

As throughout much of rural Indonesia (and indeed throughout much of rural Asia as a whole), the cultivation of rice in Toraja establishes a certain rhythm and direction to life. In most areas there is not enough accessible river flow to insure year-round cultivation, as in Bali and parts of Java. Instead, cultivation is dependent on the annual monsoon rains, which usually begin around October and continue through March or April. During the months that rains are saturating and filling the terraced fields, women grow rice seedlings and then laboriously transplant them by hand to the surrounding fields. Men by hand and buffalo plow the fields in preparation for planting, and then spend hours weeding and protecting seedlings from birds and other pests once they have taken root. They also spend countless hours and days repairing and maintaining the terracing of the fields. Both men and women hand cut and harvest the rice once it begins to mature, towards the end of the rainy season and the beginning of the dry. While children in these areas now spend a good portion of their day in school, they too are often engaged in agricultural activities of one kind or another or in the household activities that either support or result from agricultural work.

Toraja households tend to be nuclear in structure, consisting of married or unmarried couples and their children. As households mature and develop, children leave to marry and form their own household units. The older couples or single parents left behind may then begin to adopt or foster some of their grandchildren or other children to provide household labor and companionship. Or, if they are old enough or infirm enough, they may themselves be folded into a child's household. From the point of view of a person's sense of well-being, it is the household unit that provides many of the good things in life: relative safety and nurturance, relatively relaxed intimacy, and refuge from the demands and uncertainties of life outside the household. Indeed, traditional ancestral houses, called *tongkonan,* are symbolically consti- tuted as womb-like structures that are thought to be founts of fertil- ity and prosperity. Activities outside the household, on the other hand, nearly always have a more mixed valence. For example, the people Jane Wellenkamp and I worked with in the 1980s were very accomplished farmers and gardeners, but they were also quick to note that manual labor was exhausting, could cause lasting injury or premature aging, and was a primary cause of personal and social suffering. Life outside the household also exposed people to potential social dangers, such as unwanted or unfair requests for aid and assistance and black magic. Of course relations with "outside" people could also be pleasurable, as when groups of men or women or children gather to gossip and joke, or when people are able to enhance their pride and prestige by slaugh- tering animals at communal feasts. But even these enjoyable activities could turn sour.

One of the reasons the social terrain outside the household can be so treacherous to navigate is that it is organized hierarchically. As through- out much of Indonesia, in Toraja, social rank is inherited through one's family as well as achieved through one's own accomplishments, such as completing higher levels of education, holding certain kinds of jobs, or slaughtering animals at community feasts. Distinctions are drawn among traditional nobles, the newly wealthy, and commoners, and there is an elaborate etiquette to insure that each group receives the def- erence and respect it deserves. Cross-cutting this pronounced social hi- erarchy is an ethos of reciprocity in which those with more are expected to nurture and come to the assistance of those with less. In practice, higher- status and wealthy people are expected to help the lower-status and the poor with their material needs, and in return, the lower-status and the poor are expected to shower the high-status people with defer- ence and labor. If people misjudge the social terrain in some way, if they fail to give deference when deference is expected, if they fail to give as- sistance when it is warranted or if they ask for assistance when it is not, they may shame or anger others and so open themselves to retaliation in the form of reciprocal disrespect or magical attack.

The fine balancing act between giving to others what they deserve and getting from others what is one's own due comes to a high-stakes head in the meat division at community feasts. It is there when a fam- ily's rank becomes most visible and obvious to others, symbolized in a very concrete way by the amount and kind of meat it receives. It is a site where if all goes well and one receives the meat that is one's due, one leaves feeling proud, respected, and acknowledged by the community.

But if not, one can feel shamed and humiliated in front of the whole community.

Navigation of the social terrain varies by gender as well. Generally speaking, the status of women in Toraja is high: the kinship system is bilateral; women can inherit land and property; there is no preference for male children; women's work (gardening, planting, harvesting, cooking, childcare) is valued; and, from a cross-cultural point of view, gender differences are not given much cultural elaboration. For example, the Toraja language does not have separate pronouns for males and females, and the terms for siblings and grandparents are gender neutral. Further, adolescent initiation practices are relatively unelaborated, and they do not serve to highlight dramatic differences between males and females. Indeed, some prominent male roles are closely identified with feminine functions and characteristics—for example, the traditional male leader and coordinator of rice-growing activities and rituals is called the *Indo' Pandang*, literally, "Mother of the Ground" (Hollan and Wellenkamp 1994, 88–91).

Yet there is nearly complete segregation by gender in public places such as feasts and rituals, where men are given preferred food, drink, and seating. Beginning in childhood, males are given more freedom to explore the social terrain. Boys are more often encouraged to tend buffalo, gardens, and rice fields that take them away from the village, whereas girls are more often encouraged to stay closer to home to help out with childcare and other household work. By adolescence, boys are free to wander in search of romance and adventure, whereas girls are expected to travel in groups or with chaperons, especially at night. Women who try to evade these restraints on their behavior are said to deserve whatever might befall them, including rape.

While expectations for men and women vary, their roles and responsibilities are thought to be complementary. A well-functioning, prosperous household is one in which both male and female work is being performed. From a Toraja perspective, men and women need one another. Unmarried or unattached people are anomalous and are thought worthy of pity or compassion.

Age is another factor that affects how one navigates the social terrain in Toraja. Generally speaking, children and old people are given more freedom and behavioral license than young and middle-aged adults (Hollan and Wellenkamp 1996). Although people remember times as children when they were overwhelmed by learning or mastering new skills and responsibilities, most say childhood is one of the happiest periods of life, a time when other people are responsible for feeding them and they are relatively free to go to school and play with their friends. Adulthood, on the other hand, is considered to be one of the most difficult, stressful periods of life. Adults are ultimately responsible for feeding and caring for themselves *and* everyone else in the village, including their children and older, infirm parents. They also shoulder primary responsibility for maintaining the family's status and prestige by slaughtering animals at community feasts and for paying for their children's education—demands that are often at odds with one another. Given all the stresses and burdens of adulthood, many people say they look forward to old age when, like children, other people assume more responsibility for them and they have less work and worries. Older people are also freer to challenge or defy accepted rules of conduct, for example, by becoming more openly ill tempered or impatient.

Spiritual and religious beliefs and practices not only constitute an important part of the social terrain in Toraja but also affect how one maneuvers through it. Before the Dutch introduced Christianity to the highlands in the early 1900s, the Toraja followed a number of prescriptions, prohibitions, and ritual practices meant to keep them on good terms with a variety of gods, spirits, and ancestral figures. These numinous beings were thought to reward proper behavior with prosperity while punishing improper behavior with illness and misfortune. Although the vast majority of the Toraja now consider themselves to be Christian and no longer follow many of the rituals and prohibitions of their forebears, many still adhere to the general idea that spiritual beings, including God, Jesus, and ancestral figures, punish misbehavior and reward good. For the Toraja, part of being well is knowing that one has not done anything to warrant spiritual retribution.

Thus the socialscape of well-being in the Toraja countryside is not flat or uniform. One is not merely well or unwell. Rather, one moves through a dense, contoured set of culturally structured, though constantly changing, relationships and activities with both positive and negative valences. How one encounters and reacts to this socialscape will vary depending upon one's age, gender, social and marital status, wealth, occupation, level of education, type and degree of religious belief, and so on, but also by the nature of one's past experiences. To illustrate this, let us consider a day in the life of Nene'na Tandi, one of my primary informants and collaborators.

A Toraja Selfscape

At the time I knew Nene'na Tandi in the 1980s, he was approximately sixty years old and lived in a two-room bamboo thatched house with his wife and a young, adopted son. In his youth, he had attended school through grade six and had traveled as far as Irian on the west coast of New Guinea in search of employment, but had eventually returned to the highlands when he failed to acquire the wealth and prosperity he had hoped for. Since then, he had lived as a farmer and gardener in the village. Though of commoner birth, he was wickedly witty and intelligent, and his oratory skills gave him far more influence in the village than he otherwise deserved, given his middle-level family status and limited wealth.

Nene'na Tandi began most of his days by getting up at dawn and eating leftover rice and hot tea or coffee with his wife and son. As I have suggested, most Toraja enjoy these moments with family. Away from the prying eyes of neighbors and nonfamily, they can slip out of some of the etiquette that binds them in other contexts, and they are free not to worry so much about where they fit into the pronounced social hierarchy of the village. But Nene'na Tandi enjoyed these moments, particularly with his wife, even more than most because his two previous marriages had been loveless and contentious. His present wife, on the other hand, was one of his favorite companions—although such intimacy between spouses was considered highly unusual. Thus Nene'na Tandi's sense of domestic well-being derived part of its emotional force and saliency from its implicit and explicit comparison to similar but unhappy experiences in his past.

Nene'na Tandi also enjoyed being with his adopted son, one of several children he had fostered over the years, who performed much of the household's work. But the boy's presence was also a daily reminder that he himself had never been able to have children, which was embarrassing for him, because it implied that he was probably infertile, and frightening, since childlessness was thought to be one of the signs that a person was being punished by spiritual forces. Nene'na Tandi took seriously the idea that he might be worthy of retribution since he had often defied his parents and elders during his youth. Thus, the same cultural and emotional space that afforded Nene'na Tandi moments of safety and intimacy also led him to worry about the state of his spiritual health and well-being.

Even at age sixty, Nene'na Tandi would leave his house early in the morning to work in his gardens and rice fields. Whether or not he enjoyed these movements through the village and surrounding countryside depended very much on whom he encountered there. When Nene'na Tandi was with close family or friends, I often found him regaling them with his wit and charm. He could be a highly sociable man and loved to brag that since he was not wealthy, his true gifts to people were his "sweet words" and sage advice.

But as a long-time leader in the community and as someone who was concerned with maintaining his own status and prestige, he had also gotten himself involved, or had been drawn into, a number of disputes with people. As one of the first committed Christians in the community, he sometimes criticized more traditional people for their backward, superstitious ways. As a community leader, he had strong ideas about how the community should invest its resources and how it should deal with the local and national governments. As a commoner, he was resentful of those who had inherited their wealth and prestige and the advantages it gave them in acquiring even more renown through the competitive slaughter of animals at feasts. And as a former adjudicator of disputes, he had upset and alienated as many petitioners as he had rewarded or made happy.

This history of contentious relationships put Nene'na Tandi at risk, or so he thought, since it was common knowledge that people who believe themselves shamed or mistreated might use magic to retaliate. Indeed, he claimed that he had already been the victim of magic twice before in his life: once when someone from a neighboring village poisoned his palm wine in retaliation for his involvement in a divorce case, and once when a stranger, for some unknown reason, cast a spell on him as he was returning home from the market town of Rantepao. As a result of such experiences, Nene'na Tandi had acquired special medicine to protect himself from magical attack, and he would attempt to avoid unexpected meetings with strangers or people he'd had disagreements with—although such chance, unexpected meetings did sometimes occur. Thus encounters with people outside the household could undermine Nene'na Tandi's sense of well-being as well as enhance it, depending on who the people were and the nature of the encounter.

Once out in the fields or gardens, Nene'na Tandi felt relatively safe and secure, though he often complained about how exhausting the work was. If people were around, they were almost always his friends or neighbors. By late morning or midday, his son or wife would bring him a meal, and he would eat, chew betel nut, and relax for a while. If his meal and rest strengthened him, he would continue working in the fields for the remainder of the day. If, on the other hand, his food exacerbated his stomach ailments, as it sometimes did, he would return to the village at midday, forced to consider yet again whether the spirits or ancestors might have found reason to make him sick.

The return to the village at the end of the day was the reverse of the journey out: Nene'na Tandi exposed himself to possible insult or injury when away from his house or fields, but assured himself of relative safety and security once he had returned home. Once home, he usually ate his evening meal with his wife and son, and then slept with them on the floor of the back room. Sleep and dreaming could itself be eventful and expose one to yet other adventures and potential risks and dangers, since the Toraja believe that a dreamer's soul may wander away from the body during sleep and encounter other souls and spirits. Some of these encounters in dreams are thought to be prophetic: a spirit or ancestor figure gives something or takes something away, presaging either fortune or misfortune in waking life. Nene'na Tandi has had several dreams in which his deceased parents came to him offering advice and guidance, foreshadowing a positive turn of events for him. He converted to Christianity permanently only after his wife's aunt had had a dream suggesting he would die unless he immediately became a Christian.

One of the reasons Nene'na Tandi felt very paternal towards one of the boys in his hamlet was because he and the spirit of the boy's mother had had frequent sexual encounters in his dreams. Because of that, he had become convinced that he was the boy's true father. Such a conviction, and the dreams upon which it is based, allow Nene'na Tandi to believe that at least his dream spirit is capable of having children, which is comforting to him. For the Toraja, waking and dreaming consciousnesses are woven together. Events and concerns of the day can find their way into dreams. But just as certainly, dream experiences at night affect how one interprets daily events, and so one's conscious sense of well-being.

Nene'na Tandi's selfscape does and does not resemble others in Toraja. In some ways, his concerns about magical retaliation are similar to those of wealthy and high-status people, afraid of the envy and malice of those less well to do, even though he was not particularly wealthy or high status himself. This is because his charisma and oratory skills give him an influence and position he did not otherwise deserve. But note how the same gift both enhances his well-being, by improving his social status, and undermines it, by presenting him with worries and concerns other people do not have. Like other commoners, he embraces Christianity, in part, to develop a source of pride and dignity for himself apart from those controlled by the elite. And as a male, he enjoys freedom of movement throughout the socialscape and preferential consumption of valued commodities such as meat, alcohol, and tobacco, especially in public.

His relationship with his wife, his adopted son, and the dream spirit of a neighboring woman are more unique, however. And here too, the emotional valence is mixed. On the one hand, these relationships remind him of his possible infertility, and stir up guilt about his misbehavior as a youth and concerns that he is worthy of spiritual retribution. Yet the same misfortune is partially responsible for his deep (and unusual) love of his present wife, who has remained faithful and loyal to him despite the lack of children, for the satisfaction he has received from fostering a number of children over the years, and for the pleasure he derives from imagining himself as the spiritual father of a beautiful young woman's son. This illustrates that well-being or its lack for any particular individual is influenced both by that person's placement within a culturally structured social world (his or her status, gender, age, religion, and so on) and by the way his or her earlier life experiences and memoryscapes come to affect how later life events are interpreted and reacted to. For example, Tominaa Sattu, a man who shared many of Nene'na Tandi's social characteristics, often dreamed not of having sex with the spirits of beautiful young women, but of the spirits of his beloved and much-missed parents, both of whom died while he was still a boy. Now a father and grandfather himself, he often still refers to himself as an "orphan." Here is a man whose sense of well-being was deeply shaken by the loss of his parents in childhood, never to be regained completely. And Indo'na Sapan endures the embarrassment and disadvantages of being a single mother, not because she has not had the opportunity to remarry (several men have asked her), but because she refuses ever to be hurt again in the way her former husband hurt her by having affairs with other women. Her singleness compromises the well-being of her and her children in very real, significant ways, but in her mind, not so much as it would be compromised by having a husband cheat on her again.

Discussion and Conclusion

Even this abbreviated description of a day in the life of Nene'na Tandi illustrates that the ebb and flow of his sense of well-being is a function of his location in a specific cultural space, the time of day or night, his proximity or distance from specific individuals with whom he shares specific relationship histories, the degree to which he has internalized certain cultural beliefs and practices (and not others), and his memoryscapes of past experiences. And he is not unique in this regard. Other Toraja experience similar ebbs and flows in their well-being, as do all people.

We could, of course, attempt to average out this emotional flow and say, "on balance, these cultural beliefs, practices, and artifacts promote well-being while these do not." But that would be an artificial and problematic exercise. For one thing, it would ignore the very thing the self-system has evolved to capture: the flow, particularity, and epigenetic nature of life experience for a given individual. For another, it would obscure the fact that states of wellness and unwellness are always in dynamic relationship to one another, and it is this dynamic interplay that should be the focus of our studies. By virtue of valuing and rewarding certain kinds of routines and activities, all communities necessarily disvalue other kinds, thereby creating gradients of well-being that are inescapable. Ruth Benedict (1934) pointed this out long ago when she noted that what is considered "abnormal" is always relative to what is considered normal. While some communities, no doubt, are much better about minimizing states of unwellness than others, no community can eliminate them altogether. No group of people can be completely well or unwell.

I have argued that being well is a contingent, dynamic state of being that is related to fluctuating states of body and world and the interactions between the two. This dynamism should make us wary of too quickly assessing the costs and benefits of the mere existence of particular cultural beliefs and practices without first understanding when and to what degree they are enacted, with whom, under what circumstances, and the nature of their historical development. For example, because of a rebellious youth, Nene'na Tandi takes ideas about spiritual punishment more seriously than many other Toraja do, and the relatively deep internalization of these beliefs has affected his well-being in complicated ways. On the one hand it has engendered considerable fear and anxiety in him, and very likely has contributed to or exacerbated his lifelong stomach ailments. Yet it is also one of the reasons he has now become a mature, thoughtful adult who commands the respect of many of his fellow villagers. Thus current states of well-being actually may be dependent on having passed through previous periods of not being well, and conversely, current states of unwellness may have less to do with contemporary practices than with those that shaped earlier life experiences and memoryscapes.

Here again, Nene'na Tandi is not alone. We cannot assess how routines and practices affect the wellness or lack of wellness for people without also assessing how they are encountered and experienced by specific individuals over time. People do not encounter the world as blank slates; rather, their experience of the world unfolds epigenetically. What they have experienced in the past affects how they experience things in the present and future, for good or ill, for wellness or unwellness. This is an area of study that deserves much more cross-cultural research. How do societies and communities around the world "prime" people for wellness or unwellness in childhood and then later in life? Are all forms of resilience culturally specific or are there certain kinds of activities and engagements that seem to promote well-being everywhere? And how and why do activities or engagements that promote well-being for most people turn sour for others? Why is it that some Americans use competitive strategies learned and embraced in childhood to further their sense of well-being throughout the life course, whereas others learn to shun such strategies or use them in ways that alienate them from others or undermine their happiness?

I argue that studies of well-being should embrace these complexities rather than deny them or sweep them into overly static analytical categories. To admit that states of well-being are subjective and both temporally and spatially dependent does not prevent them from being studied using traditional anthropological methods. As I have suggested, we can use participant observation and perhaps certain neurological and physiological tests to examine how selfscapes ebb and flow through the course of the day and night and other culturally relevant cycles of experience. For example, we could measure stress hormone flows throughout the course of a day and night. Eventually, we might be able to collect brain scan images throughout the course of a naturally occurring day and night.

And we can use person-centered, open-ended interviews (Levy and Hollan 1998) to examine how these fluctuating states of the self-system are related to people's representations and constructions of their past experience. The latter type of engagement is essential. At bottom, wellness and unwellness are what they are felt and experienced to be, not what they appear to be from a third-person point of view. Overt behaviors and routines alone can be misleading. A routine or behavior that looks "healthy" from the outside might be practiced to avoid shame or to expiate a conscious or nonconscious sense of guilt, either one of which, over the long run, could produce depression, anxiety, and other forms of unwellness. Conversely, a behavior that appears to be unhealthy, painful, or overly taxing might be a person's way, either consciously or nonconsciously, of attempting to identify with a beloved or respected parent, mentor, or hero figure, thereby, over the long run, promoting resilience and well-being. We can know these things only by asking people about their life experiences and by exploring with them how they have learned to link and associate past and present.

By collecting and mapping the selfscapes of representative samples of people through both space and time, we can begin to build up an empirically grounded understanding of how states of well-being and dysphoria are distributed within and across culturally constituted worlds. We might then begin a comparative analysis of such mappings, looking for similarities in the ways people construct well-being as well as taking note of the ways these constructions differ. This would lead to much better understandings of what kinds of early life experiences are most likely to promote or undermine well-being at later stages of life; how variables such as gender, age, ethnicity, and religious belief and practice intersect to promote or undermine well-being; and how states of wellness and unwellness can be related to one another. Almost all societies, for example, use shame, anxiety, fear, and other unpleasant emotional states to motivate the performance of socially valued roles and behaviors (Spiro 1965). How do different societies manage the trade-off between short-term pain and long-term gain? At what point does the short-term pain, carried forward through memory and emotional association into the future, undermine the possibility of being well, and how do societies assess (or not assess) this?

Such empirically grounded work is painstaking and difficult, but it is one of the ways we can assure ourselves that our assessments of others' well-being tell us more about *them* than about our own values and moral commitments.

References

Benedict, Ruth. 1934. *Patterns of Culture*. Boston, MA: Houghton Mifflin.

Damasio, Antonio R. 1994. *Descartes' Error: Emotion, Reason, and the Human Brain*. New York: Avon Books.

———. 1999. *The Feeling of What Happens: Body and Emotion in the Making of Consciousness*. New York: Harcourt Brace.

Hallowell, A. Irving. 1955. *Culture and Experience*. Philadelphia: University of Pennsylvania Press.

Hinton, Alex, ed. 1999. *Biocultural Approaches to the Emotions*. Cambridge: Cambridge University Press.

Hollan, Douglas. 2000. "Constructivist Models of Mind, Contemporary Psychoanalysis, and the Development of Culture Theory." *American Anthropologist* 102: 538–50.

———. 2001. "Developments in Person-Centered Ethnography." In *The Psychology of Cultural Experience*, ed. Holly Mathews and Carmella Moore, 48–67. New York: Cambridge University.

———. 2004. "Self Systems, Cultural Idioms of Distress, and the Psycho-Bodily Consequences of Childhood Suffering." *Transcultural Psychiatry* 41: 62–79.

Hollan, Douglas W. and Jane C. Wellenkamp. 1994. *Contentment and Suffering: Culture and Experience in Toraja.* New York: Columbia University Press.

————. 1996. *The Thread of Life: Toraja Reflections on the Life Cycle.* Honolulu: University of Hawaii Press.

Levy, Robert I. and Douglas W. Hollan. 1998. "Person-Centered Interviewing and Observation in Anthropology." In *Handbook of Methods in Cultural Anthropology*, ed. H. Russell Bernard, 214–37. Walnut Creek, CA: Altamira Press.

Schwartz, Theodore. 1978. "Where is the Culture? Personality as the Distributive Locus of Culture." In *The Making of Psychological Anthropology*, ed. George D. Spindler, 419–41. Berkeley: University of California Press.

Spiro, Melford E. 1965. "Religious Systems as Culturally-Constituted Defense Mechanisms." In *Context and Meaning in Anthropology*, 100–13. New York: Free Press.

11

WELL-BEING AND SUSTAINABILITY OF DAILY ROUTINES
Families with Children with Disabilities in the United States

Thomas S. Weisner

Introduction

Parents everywhere have a common project: to construct a social ecology that balances what they want for themselves and their family, with what is possible given their circumstances. This project involves *sustaining* a daily routine of life. Sustainability is a holistic conceptualization of how families are doing with respect to this project. Ecological-cultural (hereafter *ecocultural*) theory suggests that sustaining a daily routine is a universal adaptive problem for all families (Whiting 1976, 1980; Munroe, Munroe, and Whiting 1981; Whiting and Edwards 1988; Weisner 1984, 1993). Ecocultural family theory uses Super and Harkness' notion of a developmental niche for the child (1980, 1986), extended to the study of the family and ecological context (Weisner 1997). Well-being is created and experienced within this cultural learning environment.

Assessing this project for families and in research in human development requires that we include the goals of parents in a community, since those goals matter for what is considered normative, and what is the appropriate moral direction for family life and development (LeVine, Miller, and West 1988). Yet assessments of families and children are too often based on the implicit or explicit adoption by researchers of goals for families and for children that come from the United States and Western Europe. For example, American parents worry if their children are not talking early; parents conflate verbal skills with intelligence, and may seek help for this developmental "delay." The goal of academic achievement and success translates into parental concerns over one milestone, but not others.

Signs of nurturance and interpersonal obligation in a young child might make many American parents concerned over insufficient independence in their child, rather than seen as a positive sign of precocious interdependence. Indeed autonomy, or the individuation part of all development, is commonly confounded with egoistic independence. Autonomy includes volitional action and agency in the service of goals (including relational and interdependent action). The goal of social intelligence and empathy in children is altogether more important in many communities than it is in the US. Such differences in the interpretations of family and child development illustrate that diverse goals and beliefs regarding what should mark a culturally constituted successful social career influence what is viewed as positive, normative development. Children are learning to be appropriate social persons, and individual, discrete measures of ability taken out of context do not capture this project. LeVine (2003) conceptualizes enculturation as the acquisition of "local idioms" based on goals and practices within diverse local populations. These local idioms (meanings, beliefs, scripts for action, shared practices, ways of organizing everyday routines of life) matter for how families sustain family life and how they conceive of and socialize for well-being in their local cultural learning environment.

What is the connection between sustainability of a meaningful routine of daily life, and well-being? Sustainability of life in a family or community grounds well-being in everyday activities, includes the goals and moral direction of life, and provides a definition that can apply cross-culturally. More sustainable routines are undoubtedly associated with well-being in that community. Well-being, in ecocultural theory, is *engaged participation in everyday cultural activities that are deemed desirable by a community, and the psychological experiences produced by such engagement.*

What constitutes a more sustainable routine of daily life that enhances well-being? The image of contexts, activities, and practices as stepping stones along a path is a useful one. Think of a daily routine as a linked set of these activities that we "step into," or engage with, as we move through the day, week, month, and years. The path exists in some local community, and intersects with many other paths. Sustainability, like well-being as I define it, must always be understood as a project somewhere in a cultural learning environment, in some particular community with its constellation of goals and local constraints and opportunities.

Sustaining a daily routine involves four processes (Weisner 2002; Weisner et al. 2005): fitting the routine to family resources, balancing varied family interests and conflicts, meaningfulness of family activities with respect to goals and values, and providing stability and predictability of the daily routine. Routines that have better resource fit, less conflict, more balance, more meaningfulness, and enough predictability are posited to be better for families, and so to provide greater well-being for those participating in them. Sustainability in the life of a family and children is better for a child's development and for parenting. To the extent that these features of a sustainable routine can be assessed and understood in a community, these data would constitute evidence for a reliable and valid contextual universal for comparing families and communities across cultures.

This is the conceptual and empirical connection between sustainability and the topic of this volume, well-being. Well-being, like sustainability, is an ongoing project, not a one-time end point. It is contextual, embedded in an everyday routine of life, and so part of some local social context with its local idioms. It includes both the local resources and ecology of the family and community, and the goals, values, and meanings that the community affords and people bring to their practices. For this reason, understanding well-being requires contextual and ethnographic data and methods, just as sustainability does.

The unit of analysis (local practices and activities) of both sustainability and well-being is very familiar and congenial to ethnographic methods, as well as to other methods anthropologists use, such as interviews, questionnaires, individual assessments, and systematic behavior observations. Activities have features that recur and structure them, including a *script* for normative conduct; *goals and values* organizing the meaning and direction of the activity; a *task* and functional outcomes the activity is there to accomplish; *people* and their relationships that are present in the activity; the motivations and feelings that people have in the setting that influence their *engagement* in it; and the *resources* needed to constitute the activity and make it happen (Cole 1996; Weisner 2002). Sustainability, because it defines a higher-quality family daily routine (which consists of activities prevalent in a community) should enhance well-being.

Sustainability of family routines differs from stress, coping, and similar challenges, although those familiar constructs are also certainly involved in sustaining a family daily routine. The stress and coping models begin with an unusual, difficult perturbation that is a challenge or threat (or at least potentially so), and then look for the responses of individuals or families to those perturbations. Resilience or adaptation is the successful response to such threats. Sustainability, however, captures another, more enduring project: juggling ongoing demands in the service of meeting long-term goals (Gallimore, Bernheimer, and Weisner 1999). Sustainability focuses on the everyday accommodations made in a local context that keep life going, that is, keep alive the daily routines expectable and meaningful in that community. Sustaining a daily routine can be positive as well as negative at times in terms of

one's affective experience and effort. Accommodations are not necessarily stressful or the result of coping with difficulty, and can be rather
unremarkable and mundane to those doing them—yet no less sustaining and promotive of well-being, often because of this everyday, implicit aspect.

Cultural goals and meanings do not simply float in a collective
community's beliefs, and then—somehow—lead to motivated actions
that can enhance well-being. Cultural models include scripts for action in settings. These scripts and the settings they are activated in then
give cultural models their "directive force" (Quinn and Holland 1987;
D'Andrade and Strauss 1992) by shaping action and thought. There is
a script for eating a meal together, attending a class, visiting grandparents, or caring for a sibling. Sustaining a daily routine that is meaningful with respect to at least some of a person's goals includes enacting a
script for these activities, which directs behavior. Enacting these scripts
are a part of what makes life worth living.

Sustainability and well-being foreground the interconnection between mind and context, and emphasize the social character of mind.
Being in a local context produces psychological experiences in individual minds. It is also of course true that individual minds vary in the
ways they appraise and experience a context. The point for thinking
about well-being in this way is that the psychological experiences are
not only *individual* intrapsychic experiences; they are a product of social
context and the "social mind" as well.

Well-being and sustainability are contextual universals: the features
of sustainability should enhance well-being in any community, but the
local meanings and contexts of that community are a part of measuring
and understanding well-being. Cultural and ethnographic studies of
well-being thus can provide evidence for universals as well as differences and particulars.

Connections of Sustainability and
Well-Being to Chapters in This Volume

Although Thin, in chapter 1, suggests that anthropology has focused
too little on well-being and positive affects and too much on adaptation,
relativism, or ill-being, students of culture and human development in
anthropology have given much more attention to positive child development and well-being than perhaps have other fields in anthropology. The comparative and analytical attention to well-being certainly
deserves renewed attention in anthropology, but Thin underestimates
the field of psychological anthropology and the study of childhood and

parenting as a rich, extensive, and long-standing research area interested in these topics (LeVine 2007). If there is one finding that is central in the field of culture and human development, it is that communities vary in what good development is, and in the ways parents and communities set children on those desired pathways. Anthropologists also recognize the universal requirements of maturation and care as important everywhere. Add the ethnographic attention to local idioms for care and parenting in these diverse cultural learning environments, ecocultural context, and everyday routines of life for children and parents, and it is evident that the study of child and family well-being in this field of anthropology is central.

Sustainability provides a link—a "translational definition"—connecting many of the anthropological perspectives on well-being featured in this volume (Weisner 1998). The essays in this volume develop, in their own ways, the features of sustainability (resources and their match to goals and values people feel they can attain, meaning and emotional experience and engagement with community practices, the benefits of low conflict and social relationships, and predictability and adaptability).

Mathews and Izquierdo emphasize in their conclusion health, sociality, existential, and structural bases of well-being. They and many other authors emphasize the importance of the experience and conceptions of well-being in particular local contexts. Izquierdo's rich ethnographic understanding of Matsigenka well-being (chapter 3) contrasts physiological health indicators (which show improvement) with the sense of community fragmentation and existential crisis in the face of the absence of a meaningful account of why distressful events are happening (all getting worse). The resources and wealth from the presence of outsiders and natural gas extraction create social conflicts that reduce well-being.

Several papers show the importance of cultural meaning and local idioms for well-being. Clark, in chapter 9, focuses on bathing in Japan, and Clark's pleasure context (settings, activities, and meanings of seeking a positive experienced state) is a rich example of a practice that enhances well-being. Mathews in chapter 8 emphasizes the meaning system of what makes life worth living in Japan, Hong Kong, and the US, as a key to the existential meanings of personal well-being. Cultural framing, social negotiations, and institutional channels all are key dimensions for creating and accounting for well-being.

Derné in chapter 6 focuses on subjective experience and the internal state of mind crucial to well-being among middle-class, upper-caste Hindu men; love itself follows from social expectations about marriage as being based on a fit with extended family life. Nurturing others (as contrasted with individual achievement as a cultural goal and self-ideal) engages experiences of well-being for these men. A cultural model leads to a script for action in this community, which in turn leads to well-being as locally defined. Heil in chapter 4 also finds that well-being in an Australian Aboriginal community involves a person's capacity to make and meet the requirements of kin-related, socially engaged responsiveness, rather than individualized physical or mental states. Adelson in chapter 5 describes the historic identification of Eastern Cree well-being with connections to their ancestral land and the cultural and familial meanings that flowed from that. Hollan in chapter 10 describes individual selfscapes, in which well-being is a subjective, temporally and spatially dependent experience. Selfscapes emerge out of a constant mapping of a person's cultural representations of past experiences onto the current culturally constituted world.

Adaptive potential is the key organizing concept in Colby's model (chapter 2); sustaining a daily routine is also an adaptive and functional project. Jankowiak in chapter 7 proposes a connection between well-being, social engagement, and a sense of personal choice: if people feel some sense of control over resources and social relationships, and have at least some of the resources to attain some of those chosen goals, they are going to feel a greater sense of well-being. Jankowiak's model emphasizes the fit between engagement and well-being: activities in a community that are not deemed desirable (or around which there is ambivalence and conflict), such as the Chinese communist-era settings without a sense of control, will not have high engagement and so will have at best mixed effects on positive well-being.

Other Indicators of Well-Being

As Colby, Thin, Jankowiak, Mathews, and Izquierdo point out, the social sciences are hardly unaware of well-being. There are extensive and well-researched empirical indices of life satisfaction, life quality, and well-being already available. These other indicators of well-being are not likely to be replaced by anthropological ones, nor should they be. There are good indicators available for child and family well-being, for instance. Brown (1997) reviews the major indicators used by the United States federal statistical system for assessing child well-being. None are existential or deeply contextual, nor do they include the moral direction and meanings important to anthropologists (except insofar as they assume that the current United States provides implicitly universal standards), but many surely matter for well-being. The indicators include child health, education, economic security, family and demographic characteristics (race, immigration, social isolation, household, and neighborhood), and social development and problem behavior indicators (such as having friends, life goals, and the universally negative consequences of chronic aggression and violence).

UNICEF (1997) collects and publishes indices on children's well-being as well. Their list includes mortality, adult literacy, GNP, nutrition, public health, education, demographic indicators (death rates, life expectancy), economic indicators, and status of women, as well as the rates of progress on each of these indicators. Bornstein et al. (2003) focus on positive development: resilience, successful adaptation, happiness, good health, and similar indicators, measured across the life span. Sutcliffe (2001) recasts many such indicators of life quality and well-being. He illuminates the stark and in some cases growing global inequality between nation-states as well as inequality among subgroups within a nation-state. Vleminckx and Smeeding (2001) provide indicators for the developed world that also show clear differences across modern nation-states. Their work provides strong evidence that the developed world is far from homogenous on a variety of indicators of life quality and well-being, and that we need to be cautious and specific when making global comparisons between the developed and the rest of the world on well-being, using conventional indicators. Anthropological perspectives on well-being will certainly add to the evidence for the need for pluralism in measuring and comparing well-being around the world.

Ben-Arieh and Goerge (2005) have assembled a rich collection of indicators of children's well being. Their book focuses on measurement and design of well-being research, and on using social indicators like well-being to affect child and family policy. A web site, www.childindicators .com, extends the use of well-being measures in the service of effective policy and practice, and a society, the International Society for Child Indicators, has been founded to further this goal.

Many of these indicators of well-being rely on *individual* indicators and then aggregate and summarize them for nations or regions. This can lead to reifying the averages across individuals and then claiming family, community, or cultural well-being at the group level, absent evidence regarding shared meanings and practices which in fact have not been collected at family, community, or cultural levels of analysis. This is a point made in many chapters in our volume. It is not that both individual and contextual indicators are not relevant, but rather that indicators at only individual levels are insufficient.

Well-being is about a person-in-context. Context or setting-level indicators are important for assessing and understanding well-being, along with individual measures. Earls and Carlson (1995) have called for the incorporation of the experiences of parents and children in local cultural context into family and child well-being work. Sustainability of family routines is a general, meaningful outcome for families that meet this criterion.

Sustainability complements other indices of well-being; it does not replace them. Sustainability and the other anthropologically informed ideas in this volume are conceptually different and add value to existing indices of quality of life and well-being. To illustrate the added value of sustainability, my collaborators and I tested whether sustainability in fact adds explanatory value alongside other indicators (both individual and context-level) of well-being and life quality. The study was of families with a child with a disability in Los Angeles. The evidence shows that a holistic assessment of sustainability in families does add both descriptive and explanatory value.

Families with Children with Disabilities in the United States

Just as for general indicators of well-being and quality of life, there already are many useful measures of well-being specific to families and children with disabilities. Hughes and Hwang (1996), for example, offer an extensive literature review of fifteen dimensions of life quality for persons with disabilities for which there are at least some validated measures and consensus within that research field (Table 11.1). These dimensions are relevant not only to individuals with disabilities and their families, but much more broadly as well. Further, these indicators include, at least indirectly, dimensions related to more existential perspectives on well-being. Many items on the list are applicable to people with disabilities cross-culturally as well, though only with the appropriate modifications, local meanings, and the addition perhaps of other indicators that matter in varied local communities (Ingstad and Whyte 1995; Skinner and Weisner 2007). I turn now to an empirical example of the use of sustainability as a holistic assessment for understanding well-being, in concert with other measures.

Families with Children with Disabilities: The CHILD Project Sample

A cohort of 102 Euro-American families with delayed children aged three to four years old was recruited into a longitudinal study in 1985–

Table 11.1 Fifteen Dimensions (Consensus Literature Review) of Quality of Life (General and for Persons with Disabilities) (Hughes and Hwang 1996)

Social relationships and interaction (friendship, responsibility, interdependence, etc.)

Psychological well-being and personal satisfaction

Employment (skills, satisfaction, characteristics, etc.)

Self-determination, autonomy, and personal choice

Recreation and leisure

Personal competence, community adjustment, and independent living skills

Residential environment

Community integration

Normalization

Support services received

Individual and demographic indicators (income, initiative, access to transportation, etc.)

Personal development and fulfillment

Social acceptance, social status, and ecological fit

Physical and material well-being

Civic responsibility (voting, etc.)

---

86 in Los Angeles, California. This is the CHILD Project sample (Gallimore et al. 1989). Parents were primarily in their early to mid-thirties when we first contacted them. Twelve percent were single mothers (due to divorce, separation, widowhood, or having never married) or in a variety of other residential and marital circumstances (e.g., living with parents). About 25 percent of the mothers were employed full-time, and families ranged from below poverty level in a number of families, to a family with income over $150,000 a year. (Further details concerning the sample, recruitment, and attrition (9 percent) are available in Gallimore et al. 1996).

Developmental Delay

Each family in our sample has a child who had been judged to be "developmentally delayed" by a professional or an agency. *Developmental delay* is a term of relatively recent vintage and lacks definitional specificity (Bernheimer and Keogh 1986). It is essentially a nonspecific "clinical" term with less ominous overtones for the future than "retarded" or "handicapped." There is considerable diagnostic ambiguity and change in diagnosis (Bernheimer and Keogh 1988; Bernheimer, Keogh, and Coots 1993).[1] Children with known genetic abnormalities were excluded from the sample because we wanted to focus on families where the future prognosis was ambiguous and uncertain. To focus the sample further, children whose delays were associated with either known prenatal alcohol or drug usage or with postnatal neglect or abuse were excluded (Bernheimer and Keogh 1986, 1982; Bernheimer, Keogh, and Coots 1993; Gallimore et al. 1996). In addition to standardized assessments on all children, we adopted a construct parents frequently used in their conversations with us: child hassle. "Hassle" is not pejorative in parents' understanding, but rather an everyday ethnopsychological term, a key word (Wierzbicka 1997) used by many parents to describe their experiences. "Hassle" describes not only the child's behavioral, medical, and socioemotional difficulties but also *the effects of those difficulties on the family routine.* Higher hassle children displayed behavior problems that were troubling to families because they had a significant impact on the daily routine.[2]

Assessment of Family Sustainability and Ecocultural Context

Sample families were visited by a trained interviewer/fieldworker at child ages 3, 7, 11, 13 and 16. These fieldworkers conducted semistructured interviews with the parents, the Ecocultural Family Interview (EFI); each interview lasted from one to three hours. Parents were encouraged to "tell their story" about their child and about how they were or were not adapting their family routine, and in response to what or whom (Bernheimer and Weisner 2007). There were no false negatives; if parents did not bring up topics, we used probes that carefully covered standard ecocultural domains (resources, supports, child services, siblings, work schedules, goals, religious beliefs, etc.). Each family also completed a questionnaire covering standard demographic information and socioeconomic status characteristics of the family. Field notes also were compiled for each family. (For additional information on the various methods used in the study, see Gallimore et al. 1993; Gallimore et al. 1996; Nihira, Weisner, and Bernheimer 1994; Weisner, Matheson, and Bernheimer 1996.)

Our fieldwork staff held a series of meetings to discuss, case by case, the nature of sustainability and well-being across the families. Qualitative assessment of each family required *contextual* knowledge about each family as well as across families; *depth* of understanding; *breadth* of knowledge about the family; and *accuracy* and *precision* about what features (such as material and social resources, family goals, or the child's behavioral problems) actually look and feel like in the context of everyday family life (Becker 1996; Weisner 1996). We attempted to develop specific indicators that would differentiate what we knew of family strengths and weaknesses within the overall framework of ecocultural theory. The typology we eventually developed emerged from dynamic discussions closely related to our comprehensive knowledge of the families and children. Fieldworkers and interviewers carefully reviewed each family, using the four criteria for assessing a daily routine (ecological and resource fit, balanced interests and conflicts, meaningfulness, and stability/predictability). Assessments were made at child ages 3, 7, 11, and 13. We also summarized the resources and constraints facing families using three indicators: socioeconomic status and resources, the family workload for accommodating to the child with disabilities, and the amount and nature of social support and connections for the family (Nihira, Weisner, and Bernheimer 1994; Weisner 1993). Fieldworkers doing assessments had no knowledge of test scores, scores on other family assessment measures, or any of the quantitative measures of family or child status.

Quality of Life

We administered the "Quality of Life Scale" (QOL) (Olson and Barnes 1982) to parents when children were age thirteen. This scale includes forty items that define twelve factors: health, marriage and family life, friends, extended family, home, education, time, religion, employment, financial well-being, impact of mass media, neighborhood, and community. Respondents are asked to indicate their satisfaction on each item using a 5-point scale, with 1 = dissatisfied and 5 = extremely satisfied.[3]

Sustainability Adds Value and Understanding

So, we have a suite of measures that all are implicated in one way or another, at least conceptually and often empirically, with understandings of well-being for children and families. This suite of measures includes the qualitative, holistic assessment of sustainability. I will briefly summarize four patterns of sustainability across families, and then consider the relationships between sustainability and some of these other measures. For example, would our qualitative construct of sustainability and well-being add value to a very comprehensive and widely used standard assessment tool such as QOL? Would the cognitive developmental assessments of each child predict sustainability?

Patterns of Family Sustainability

We identified families from low to high sustainability (Weisner et al. 2005). *Multiply Troubled* families are easy to recognize at the low sustainability end. These families led chaotic, precarious lives: few and uncertain resources, very little stability in their routines, a lot of conflict, and the lowest experience of life meeting their goals in meaningful ways. Parents sometimes had personal problems (alcoholism, mental illness, physical health) and felt overwhelmed. Their children were high hassle and more often than not had multiple problems. Fortunately, at least in our sample, there were no more than 8 percent of families in this category across our four visits. Unfortunately, there was little change over time in the low sustainability and well-being of these families.

The following case exemplifies the difficulties these families faced:[4]

> At the age 11 visit, Carolyn was a single parent, living with her son Max in a tiny apartment with no outside play space. She was still employed as a veterinarian's assistant, making $20,000 a year. She was unable to afford health insurance, but made too much money to qualify for AFDC. In addition, she was denied help from SSI because Max did not fit their eligibility criteria. His only diagnosis was "mild mental retardation." But according to Carolyn, "his behavior is so bad I can't stand being around him." His speech was largely unintelligible, and he was unable to get along with other children in or out of school.

> Carolyn had no one she could count on for help. Her mother lived nearby, but was embarrassed by her grandson, and so Carolyn refused to ask her for help. Her neighbors were unwilling to watch Max because of his behavior problems. Carolyn disapproved of them anyway—they were too rowdy, always playing loud music. The only person who helped occasionally was Carolyn's sister, who took him once in a while. Recently Carolyn's schedule was changed from Monday thru Friday to Tuesday through Saturday. She worries about being able to keep her job because of the childcare problems.

> Carolyn was pessimistic about the future. She felt the school was either unwilling or unable to teach Max anything, and she worried that the time would come when it was too late. She described herself and her son as hapless victims of an uncaring bureaucracy. When asked what she did when she felt overwhelmed, she responded, "I have to keep going. I'm by myself."

The next group, *Vulnerable but Struggling* families were "hanging on." Some 9–17 percent of families fell into this group. Parents talked about just enduring, being slow and steady, and taking things as they come. More of these parents were religious; many said that God has given them both a burden and an opportunity and they are a part of His plan (Weisner, Beizer, and Stolze 1991). Their goals and meaningfulness sometimes were strengths for them in spite of their struggles. Most had too few resources to reliably make ends meet, relatively few outside contacts, and conflicts among family members.

Improving/Resilient families were from 25–32 percent of the sample over time, and struggled as well. Things were not easy. These families had as good a fit between the resources and demands of their ecology as the High Sustainability group described below, but were likely to be dissatisfied with the often poor balance and greater conflict among different family members' goals, and the sometimes lower meaningfulness of their routines. Often the dissatisfaction could be traced in part to the hassle and problems presented by the child. One mother described her family's struggles to meet the needs of all family members—the two parents, the eleven-year-old child with delays, and a two-year-old:

> We've had a man coming to our house every week who's a psychologist and who is a behavioral specialist, and Pete isn't having any unusual behavior; he's really very normal behaviorally, but we were having such a hard time in our household trying to juggle him, how much attention he gets, how much attention for our daughter, each other, because we have very little time together. We were really having a hard time … my husband and I were just really locking horns over a lot of issues.

In spite of her statement that her son was "normal behaviorally," this mother described considerable aggression from Pete to his younger sibling. Her husband's availability also had become more limited recently; he had become extremely involved in Regional Center politics, in part as a strategy for increasing their knowledge about available services:

> My husband and I … have tried so hard to find every resource possible. … I mean almost obsessively so, he finally decided that he would just get on the board of Tri-County. We found someone who invited him to join the board. He is now on three committees and the head of one of them and very much in charge up there.

While they welcomed the additional information they gained from his activities, they were not satisfied with their family life—too much of their energy was going towards Pete, to the detriment of other family members.

Stable/Sustainable families (about 40–50 percent of the sample), with the highest sustainability scores at age eleven, have children with the lowest behavioral, medical, and communication hassle scores for any of the four groups and the fewest number of reported child problems. Jim and Ann Turner, for example, have high family sustainability and well-being. Their daughter Tori has been diagnosed with mild cerebral palsy and ADD. Though Tori has some significant disabilities, Ann does not experience these as leading to significant hassle, either behavioral, medical, or in communication, and reports relatively few child problems, and so she (as well as Jim, by Ann's report) feels that their daily routine is reasonably stable by the time Tori reaches age eleven:

> At the time of the 11-year visit, Jim and Ann reported that things were, for the most part, running smoothly. They had recently moved to a new neighborhood with more children, further away from traffic, with a large front and back yard. Anne was currently a full time homemaker, and Jim had recently returned to school to obtain his MBA, attending classes three nights a week and Saturday mornings. He continued to work full time for the phone company. Even with Jim's schedule, the Turners continued to maintain "family times." They made it a point to sit down 2–3 times a week to play a game with the children, 10-year old Tori and 13-year old Jack, or to watch a movie selected by the children. On Saturdays after his class, Jim usually worked out in the yard and the kids worked with him, giving Ann the opportunity to clean house, do laundry, etc. Every Sunday, after attending church as a family, they spent the afternoon and evening with the paternal grandparents. While Jim's schedule did cut down on his time with the kids, both parents subscribed to "quality over quantity." Thus, when there was an airfare sale, Jim took Jack to Hawaii for his birthday. "It wasn't extreme—we don't buy Nintendos or anything, and the fares were so low, we couldn't afford not to."
>
> Tori, who has mild cerebral palsy and ADD, was still in a regular classroom and continuing to struggle. All Ann wanted was for Tori to get the help she needed; she didn't care what label or diagnosis was given. Although the teacher, psychologist, and speech teacher all felt she needed resource specialist help, the resource specialist said Tori wasn't "bad enough." The Turners have requested a new IEP [Individualized Educational Plan] meeting. It wasn't even important to the Turners that Tori stay in regular education; Jim was ready to put her back in special education. In spite of her school problems, Tori has never had problems with her self-esteem. Ann attributed this to the fact that "there's no deception—she feels there's no deception about what's going on." When Tori asked why she couldn't write as well as her classmates, her mother explained it was probably because she has mild cerebral palsy, and she can't make her hands work the way she would like.
>
> At home Tori needed minimal supervision. She was able to entertain herself for long periods of time, looking at books, and working on her math and spelling on the computer, which she enjoys. Ann made it a point to monitor Tori's work. Although Tori could dress herself, she had no concept of what goes together, and Ann usually had to oversee her choices. She could put her socks on, but was still unable to tie her shoes, so Ann bought the ones with velcro fasteners. When Tori left the front yard, she had to tell her mother, but Ann was adamant that she took no more time

to supervise than any other 10-year-old. There was also less medical supervision necessary than before, as Tori's cardiac situation had stabilized, and she was only being monitored by her pediatrician.

This visit to the Turners was summarized by the fieldworker as follows: "Easy child, mild delays, heart condition still unresolved but no impact on daily routine. Familial orientation, fundamentalist religious beliefs, mother sees child as a blessing and is happy to focus all her time and energy on the family."

Sustainability Complements Other Measures and Adds Value

The assessments, scales, questionnaires, and related information our project collected on children and families proved useful; they were associated in varying degrees to the four sustainability patterns (Multiply Troubled, Vulnerable but Struggling, Improving/Resilient, and Stable/Sustainable) that we found in our qualitative analysis. But a great deal of information about family sustainability was added, unique to the qualitative groups we formed. For example, Quality of Life scores based on individual reports by mothers accounted for about 25 percent of the variation in assignment of families to the four sustainability groups—a significant contribution, but leaving a good deal more to be understood through qualitative and contextual analysis of family sustainability. QOL has twelve subscales in the overall measure, and five of the twelve (marriage and family life, friendship, employment, home, and religion) were related to sustainability. Rather than based on crisis or unusual stress, perceptions of quality of life in these families were mediated by the overall daily routine and the degree to which it is sustainable. Assessments of caregivers' QOL combined with qualitative assessments of family context jointly enhance the understanding of the impact of disability on family life over either one separately (Bernheimer and Weisner n.d.).

Although it might be thought that the child's IQ and developmental assessments would be associated with family sustainability and well-being, this was not the case. This is an important nonrelationship, since these developmental scores are often used to assess functioning levels and severity of cognitive disability in children, with the inference that the lower the scores, the lower the family well-being as well. In our sample, however, families can have higher or lower sustainability independent of these normed child assessments. But the parental folk constructs of hassle show a different picture. Families with high hassle children *were* more likely to decline in sustainability over time, while families with children with lower hassle and problems were more likely to move into the high sustainability category as the years went by. By the time the children with disabilities reached age eleven, troublesome child characteristics clearly were a hindrance to constructing a sustainable routine, just as easier child characteristics seemed to facilitate the process. In other words, there is evidence that as children get older, their *behavioral* characteristics are associated with parents' ability to sustain their family routine, but the child's *cognitive* abilities are largely unrelated. The reasons for this, based on the ethnographic data, appear to be that less child hassle and fewer child behavioral problems clearly increase the ability of parents and siblings to organize a daily routine that is lower in conflict, relatively predictable, and relatively more meaningful for all family members than is the case for high hassle and multiple-problem children. That is, those families have relatively greater well-being.

Sustainability among families with a child with disabilities shows that the construct can be reliably understood in context and rated across families. It suggests that the other complementary measures of life quality and child developmental status which we used also are useful in gaining a more holistic understanding of these families and children, and that sustainability adds significantly to our understanding of these other measures. A holistic anthropological perspective on family sustainability and well-being can, and I believe should be used wherever possible and appropriate, along with other methods and measures. In this way, the added value of including a deeper understanding of local context, cultural ecology, local idioms, and the meaning and direction of a well-lived life will enrich and extend other widely used indicators of well-being.

Notes

The research on the CHILD study was supported by National Institute of Child Health and Human Development Grants No. HD 19124 and HD No. 11944 (Ronald Gallimore, Barbara Keogh, and Weisner, PI's), and with support from the Qualitative Data & Fieldwork Laboratory, Center for Culture & Health, MRRC Core Facility, UCLA, HD011944 (Weisner, PI, Dr. Eli Lieber, co-director). Thanks to the participating children and their families who wanted their stories told, to Dr. Lucinda Bernheimer for work on the Quality of Life study, to Drs. Catherine Matheson and Jenni Coots for collaboration on the sustainability study, to colleagues in the Center for Culture and Health, Semel Neuropsychiatric Institute, and to Professors Donald Guthrie and Gwen Gordon for statistical analyses.

1. The mean developmental quotient (a normed indicator of cognitive development) for the children in our sample was 72 when the children were age three to four, and ranged from 38 to 117. Though some children improved and others declined over time, this mean level for the sample remained about the same through age eleven.
2. Interviewer ratings of child hassle used a 9-point scale of hassles/problems in everyday life, rated by fieldworkers from 0 = low to 8 = high. Hassle includes: (1) behavioral hassles (e.g., tantrums), (2) medical hassles (e.g., seizures, use of multiple medications), and (3) communicative hassles (e.g. hard to understand, nonverbal, points, grunts).
3. A total unweighted sum score ranges from 40 to 200. Overall test-retest reliability is 0.64, with Cronbach alpha 0.92.
4. All case material has been disguised by changing names and nonessential information so that no family could be identified by using the information presented.

References

Becker, Howard S. 1996. "The Epistemology of Qualitative Research." In *Ethnography and Human Development: Context and Meaning in Social Inquiry,* ed. Richard Jessor, Anne Colby, and Richard A. Shweder, 53–71. Chicago: University of Chicago Press.

Ben-Arieh, Asher and Robert M Goerge, eds. 2005. *Indicators of Children's Well Being: Understanding their Role, Usage and Policy Influence.* Dordrecht, Netherlands: Springer.

Bernheimer, Lucinda P. and Barbara K. Keogh. 1982. *Research on Early Abilities of Children with Handicaps.* (Final report, longitudinal sample). Los Angeles: University of California.

———. 1986. "Developmental Disabilities in Preschool Children." In *Advances in Special Education,* ed. Barbara K. Keogh, 5: 61–94. Greenwich. CT: JAI Press.

———. 1988. "The Stability of Cognitive Performance of Developmentally Delayed Children." *American Journal of Mental Retardation* 92: 539–42.

Bernheimer, Lucinda P. and Thomas S. Weisner. n.d. "Quality of Life for Caregivers of Children with Developmental Delays: Relationships with Child Characteristics and the Family Daily Routine." Manuscript.

———. 2007. "Let me just tell you what I do all day ...": The Family Story at the Center of Intervention Research and Practice." *Infants & Young Children* 20 (3): 192–201.

Bernheimer, Lucinda P., Barbara K. Keogh, and Jennifer J. Coots. 1993. "From Research to Practice: Support for Developmental Delay as a Preschool Category of Exceptionality." *Journal of Early Intervention* 17: 97–106.

Bornstein, Marc H., Lucy Davidson, Corey L. Keyes, and Kristin A. Moore, eds. 2003. *Well-Being: Positive Development Across the Life Course.* Mahwah, NJ: Lawrence Erlbaum Associates.

Brown, Brett V. 1997. "Indicators of Children's Well-Being: A Review of Current

Indicators Based on Data from the Federal Statistical System." In *Indicators of Children's Well-Being*, ed. Robert M. Hauser, Brett Brown, and William R. Prosser, 3–35. New York: Russell Sage.

Cole, Michael. 1996. *Cultural Psychology: A Once and Future Discipline.* Cambridge, MA: Harvard University Press.

D'Andrade, Roy and Claudia Strauss. 1992. *Human Motives and Cultural Models.* Cambridge, MA: Cambridge University Press.

Earls, Felton and Maya Carlson. 1995. "Towards Sustainable Development for American Families." *Daedalus* 122: 93–121.

Gallimore, Ronald, Lucinda P. Bernheimer, and Thomas S. Weisner. 1999. "Family Life is More than Managing Crisis: Broadening the Agenda of Research on Families Adapting to Childhood Disability." In *Developmental Perspectives on Children with High-Incidence Disabilities*, ed. Ronald Gallimore, Lucinda Bernheimer, Donald L. MacMillan, Deborah L. Speece, and Sharaon Vaughn, 55–80. Mahwah NJ: LEA Press.

Gallimore, Ronald, Thomas S. Weisner, Sandra Z. Kaufman, and Lucinda P. Bernheimer. 1989. "The Social Construction of Ecocultural Niches: Family Accommodation of Developmentally Delayed Children." *American Journal of Mental Retardation* 94 (3): 216–30.

Gallimore, Ronald, Thomas S. Weisner, Donald Guthrie, Lucinda P. Bernheimer, and Kazuo Nihira. 1993. "Family Response to Young Children with Developmental Delays: Accommodation Activity in Ecological and Cultural Context." *American Journal of Mental Retardation* 98 (2): 185–206.

Gallimore, Ronald, Jennifer J. Coots, Thomas S. Weisner, Helen Garnier, and Donald Guthrie. 1996. "Family Responses to Children with Early Developmental Delays II: Accommodation Intensity and Activity in Early and Middle Childhood." *American Journal of Mental Retardation* 101 (3): 215–32.

Hughes, Carolyn and Bogseon Hwang. 1996. "Attempts to Conceptualize and Measure Quality of Life." In *Quality Of Life, Volume I: Conceptualization and Measurement*, ed. Robert L. Schalock and Gary N. Siperstein, 51–61. Washington, DC: American Association on Mental Retardation.

Ingstad, Benedicte and Susan R. Whyte. 1995. *Disability and Culture.* Berkeley: University of California Press.

LeVine, Robert A. 2003. *Childhood Socialization: Comparative Studies of Parenting, Learning, and Educational Change.* Hong Kong: Comparative Education Research Centre.

———. 2007. "Ethnographic Studies of Childhood: A Historical Overview." *American Anthropologist* 109 (2): 247–60.

LeVine, Robert A., Patrice M. Miller, and Mary M. West, eds. 1988. *Parental Behaviors in Diverse Societies.* San Francisco: Jossey-Bass.

Munroe, Robert, Ruth Munroe, and Beatrice Whiting, eds. 1981. *Handbook of Cross Cultural Human Development.* New York: Garland STPM Press.

Nihira, Kazuo, Thomas S. Weisner, and Lucinda P. Bernheimer. 1994. "Ecocultural Assessment in Families of Children with Developmental Delays: Construct and Concurrent Validities." *American Journal of Mental Retardation* 98 (5): 551–66.

Olson, David. H. and Howard L. Barnes. 1982. *Quality of Life, Adolescent Form.* St. Paul: University of Minnesota.

Quinn, Naomi and Dorothy Holland. 1987. Introduction to *Cultural Models in Language and Thought*, 3–40. New York: Cambridge University Press.

Skinner, Debra and Thomas S. Weisner. 2007. "Sociocultural Studies of Families of Children with Intellectual Disabilities." *Mental Retardation and Developmental Disabilities Research Reviews* 13: 302–12.

Super, Charles and Sara Harkness, eds. 1980. *Anthropological Perspectives on Child Development: New Directions for Child Development*, Volume 7. San Francisco: Jossey-Bass.

Super, Charles and Sara Harkness. 1986. "The Developmental Niche: A Conceptualization at the Interface of Child and Culture." *International Journal of Behavior Development* 9: 1–25.

Sutcliffe, Bob. 2001. *100 Ways of Seeing an Unequal World*. London: Zed Books.

UNICEF. 1997. *The State of the World's Children 1997*. New York: Oxford University Press.

Vleminckx, Koen and Timothy M. Smeeding, eds. 2001. *Child Well-Being, Child Poverty and Child Policy in Modern Nations*. Bristol, UK: The Policy Press.

Weisner, Thomas S. 1984. "Ecocultural Niches of Middle Childhood: A Cross-Cultural Perspective." In *Development During Middle Childhood: The Years from Six to Twelve*, ed. W. Andrew Collins, 335–69. Washington, DC: National Academy of Sciences Press.

———. 1993. "Siblings in Cultural Place: Ethnographic and Ecocultural Perspectives on Siblings of Developmentally Delayed Children." In *Siblings of Individuals with Mental Retardation, Physical Disabilities, and Chronic Illness*, ed. Zolinda Stoneman and Phyllis Berman, 51–83. Baltimore, MD: Brooks Press.

———. 1996. "Why Ethnography Should be the Most Important Method in the Study of Human Development." In *Ethnography and Human Development: Context and Meaning in Social Inquiry*, ed. Richard Jessor, Anne Colby, and Richard Shweder, 305–24. Chicago: University of Chicago Press.

———. 1997. "The Ecocultural Project of Human Development: Why Ethnography and its Findings Matter." *Ethos* 25 (2): 177–90.

———. 1998. "Human Development, Child Well-being, and the Cultural Project of Development." In *Socio-emotional Development Across Cultures*. Vol. 81 (Fall), of *New Directions in Child Development*, ed. Dinesh Sharma and Kurt Fischer, 69–85. San Francisco: Jossey-Bass.

———. 2002. "Ecocultural Understanding of Children's Developmental Pathways." *Human Development* 45 (4): 275–81.

Weisner, Thomas S., Laura Beizer, and Lori Stolze. 1991. "Religion and the Families of Developmentally Delayed Children." *American Journal of Mental Retardation* 95 (6): 647–62.

Weisner, Thomas S., Catherine Matheson, and Lucinda P. Bernheimer. 1996. "American Cultural Models of Early Influence and Parent Recognition of Developmental Delays: Is Earlier Always Better than Later?" In *Parents' Cultural Belief Systems*, ed. Sara Harkness and Charles M. Super, 496–531. New York: Guilford Press.

Weisner, Thomas S., Catherine Matheson, Jennifer Coots, and Lucinda P. Bernheimer. 2005. "Sustainability of Daily Routines as a Family Outcome." In

Learning in Cultural Context: Family, Peers and School, ed. Ashley E. Maynard and Mary I. Martini, 47–74. New York: Kluwer/Plenum.

Whiting, Beatrice. 1976. "The Problem of the Packaged Variable." In *The Developing Individual in a Changing World: Historical and Cultural Issues*, ed. Klaus Riegel and Jack Meacham, 1: 303–9. Netherlands: Mouton.

———. 1980. "Culture and Social Behavior: A Model for the Development of Social Behavior." *Ethos* 8: 95–116.

Whiting, Beatrice and Carolyn Edwards. 1988. *Children of Different Worlds: The Formation of Social Behavior*. Cambridge, MA: Harvard University Press.

Wierzbicka, Anna. 1997. *Understanding Cultures through their Key Words*. New York: Oxford University Press.

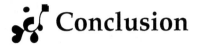 Conclusion

TOWARDS AN ANTHROPOLOGY OF WELL-BEING
Gordon Mathews and Carolina Izquierdo

As the reader is by this point no doubt well aware, the chapters of this book do not set forth a single research agenda. As we noted in the introduction, anthropological approaches to well-being are today marked by their diversity, a diversity that this book illustrates. The purpose of this book has not been to set forth a single investigative path for the anthropological study of well-being, but rather to show the variety and richness of anthropological investigations into what it means to be happy and well in different cultural contexts. This richness can serve as an empirical antidote to the straitjackets of comparison adhered to by some other disciplines, such as economics and psychology, which more or less insist on a common standard of measurement for all societies. It can also inspire students of anthropology to think about their own research in the context of well-being, and can show them an array of different modes of inquiry into the investigation of different aspects of well-being, some of which might usefully be applied to their own research.

What is of pivotal importance, then, is the singularity of the chapters in this book, reflecting the singularity of the societies they examine in their different "pursuits of happiness." Nonetheless, comparison of and conversation between these chapters may be useful in enabling a fuller understanding of the anthropological investigation of well-being in both its promise and its limitations. In this conclusion, we offer such a conversation. We begin by examining the chapters of each of this book's four sections, to see how they specifically address one another. We then draw back, to consider in a broader sense the anthropological investigation of well-being, and the ways in which individuals and societies may be compared as to well-being.

Considering and Conversing between This Book's Chapters

Let us first examine the two theoretical chapters that make up Part One. The chapters of this initial section of the book have an ambitious agenda: they seek to set forth well-being as a central concern for anthropology.

Thin in chapter 1 asks why anthropologists have not paid heed to well-being, and points out the various anthropological biases that have hindered the study of well-being. He also discusses areas of anthropology that could benefit from consideration of well-being, including "research and writing on morality, value, development, human rights, poverty, health, and mental health." His chapter, written largely from a British anthropological perspective (which may be somewhat more dismissive of the study of well-being than its American counterpart), is a call for a new kind of anthropology, one that intellectually explores morality and its complexities, and that does not shy away from moral evaluation. His argument (as well as Colby's at points) is reminiscent of that of Scheper-Hughes (1995), calling for "the primacy of the ethical" in an anthropology explicitly seeking to better the world. Calls such as these are important, but tend to leave aside the question of on what basis, exactly, moral and ethical evaluations are to be made. Who do we think we are, one might ask, making moral judgments on other peoples whose lives we cannot fully understand? Thin argues that the close intellectual examination of morality can make such judgment valid. He also implies, as Hatch (1983) argues in this book's introduction, that there are areas of human suffering—torture, rape, famine, political oppression—that are so egregious that a refusal to make moral judgment is an abdication of moral responsibility. Whether or not one follows Thin's logic—and the ethnographic chapters in this book do not generally engage in moral evaluation (although their authors' sympathies are often quite apparent)—he makes a powerful argument in his chapter, well worth wrestling with. Why study well-being across societies except to make the world a better place? And how can we make the world a better place if we deny the possibility of an objective basis upon which to evaluate the world's different societies?

If Thin's call for moral comparison and evaluation is to be heeded, then a way to measure and compare well-being is required, one that goes beyond the "soft comparison"—descriptive and largely nonevaluative—made possible through ethnography. Thin sets forth one basis for this by untangling in his chapter the semantics of and motivations for the study of well-being in anthropology, paving the way for more rigorous comparison. However, Colby in chapter 2 goes further, in arguing that a universal measure of well-being is indeed possible and desirable, and that there can indeed be "a truly objective theory of well-being."

Much of Colby's chapter involves his explication of the historical background of the anthropological study of well-being, and the logic for his comparative theory of "adaptive potential," rather than its explicit methodology and results, which he has spelled out in writings elsewhere. He discusses the problem of cultural relativism—a fundamental obstacle confronting any effort at cultural comparison—arguing that it stems from a faulty theory of culture, one that sees culture as autonomous and transcendent of individual human beings. In its place, he offers his own theory of culture as "self-world," intrinsically linked to biology. For Colby, self-world is the unit of analysis for his questionnaire measurement of adaptive potential, which he theorizes as well-being. Self-world is the logical unit for anthropological analysis, he argues, and this is the unit explicitly or implicitly used in the ethnographic chapters in this book—explicitly by Hollan in chapter 10, but implicitly by virtually every chapter.

However, the other anthropologists in this book diverge—with the partial exception of Weisner's chapter 11—from Colby's method of using survey questionnaires to get at well-being, relying instead on ethnography as the basis for their chapters. Colby fully understands the importance of ethnography, and writes that his method could be used in conjunction with and even as a guide for ethnography. But the fact remains that if Colby is right that a cross-cultural measurement of well-being is feasible and valid in its findings, then the anthropological study of well-being would be far simpler and more straightforward than it is. Indeed, if a fully valid cross-cultural measure of well-being did exist, then ethnographic portrayals of well-being might perhaps not even be necessary. Most of the authors in this book, including we who edit it, believe that statistical measures cannot substitute for ethnography. Statistical measures of well-being are not inherently flawed, but they are inherently incomplete (just as ethnographies themselves can have lacunae and interpretive idiosyncrasies). Only a detailed, on-the-ground ethnography can provide the social and cultural context without which well-being in a given society cannot be fully understood—a position with which Colby himself largely although not entirely agrees.

Thin and Colby represent one distinct type of anthropological investigation of well-being, based in the explicit moral or quantitative comparison of societies as to well-being. We have included these chapters in this book because, in any full portrayal of the anthropological treatment of well-being, approaches such as these must be recognized and seriously considered. The remainder of this book, however, has proceeded down a different path. This is a path based not in the explicit "hard" comparison of well-being in different societies, using evaluative moral judgments or cross-cultural survey data or both, but rather on the more implicit "soft" comparison of well-being afforded by ethnographic portraits placed in juxtaposition—analytic but not evaluative comparison, based more in Geertzian interpretation than on any assumption of moral or scientific objectivity. Nonetheless, it is at least possible that as quantitative measurement of complex areas of human life becomes more sophisticated, the arguments in these two chapters will be the wave of the future.[1]

The three chapters in Part Two all depict small-scale societies attempting to preserve their senses of well-being in the face of widespread encroachment by the state and the world. Each of the societies portrayed in these chapters has its own term for and conception of well-being. For the Matsigenka of the Peruvian Amazon, as depicted by Izquierdo in chapter 3, it is *shinetagantsi,* embodying "ideas and ideals of what the Matsigenka consider the basic premise of a good life." This involves little self-conscious reflection—Izquierdo's questions about personal happiness elicited only "blank stares" among the Matsigenka—but rather the ideals of providing for one's family, improving upon one's productive skills, and keeping harmonious social relations throughout a long and peaceful life. For the Aborigines of Murrin Bridge, New South Wales, as portrayed by Heil in chapter 4, it is "being well," which means "being there," thoroughly immersed in the social relations and demand sharing of one's "mob." As with the Matsigenka, it is not physical well-being—Heil's informants had little interest in talking about their diabetes, her original topic of research—but social well-being that is the essence of "being well" for the Murrin Bridge Aborigines, an active engagement in the social that they contrast with more self-oriented "whitefella ways." For the eastern James Bay Cree, as depicted by Adelson in chapter 5, it is *miyupimaatisiiun,* "being alive well," "the assertion of one's proper place in a broadly defined social and physical Cree landscape." This conception is more explicitly tied to the land than the other two concepts of well-being in this section, and it is potentially shaken by the fact that the Cree's relation to their land is changing. As they become more linked to their town and its urbanized life, *miyupimaatisiiun* may become a marker of an idealized past, Adelson speculates. With this, just as Cree conceptions of their cultural identity may change, so too may change their ideas of well-being and what it consists of.

Underlying these different conceptualizations of well-being is the fact that each of these societies has its own unique cultural context. The richness of these chapters lies in their portrayals of these contexts. These different small-scale societies, one in the jungle, one in the near-desert, and one in the Arctic, each with different kinds of relations to the society and state that surrounds it, are in a very real sense hardly comparable. But at the same time, the reader will see that there are indeed distinct commonalities of well-being in their portrayals. The three societies' indigenous concepts of well-being have broad similarities, in that they are based in kin groupings, social networks, land, and cultural values distinctly different from and at least partially opposed to those of the encroaching state and world. While we don't get enough data from these relatively brief chapters to completely understand the cultural context of these societies' senses of well-being, we do get a very solid sense of how well each of these societies is managing to preserve its well-being against the encroachments of state and world.

Indeed, a major point of comparison in these portrayals stems from their different positions in dealing with the encroachments of state and world, and the differing degrees of power they possess in preserving their autonomy. Adelson's Cree have weathered the initial onslaught of state and world, and can assert their own cultural autonomy. It is remarkable that Ted Moses, their former chief, can even assert the anthropologically sophisticated view that Cree culture is ever changing, in accordance with what the Cree themselves decide they want it to be. Izquierdo's Matsigenka, on the other hand, are in the midst of the state's and world's overwhelming cultural onslaught. They have little confidence in their future, as shown by the pessimism expressed by Izquierdo's collaborators: their belief that, despite physiological indicators to the contrary, their well-being is in decline. The Matsigenka currently also suffer from an increase in sorcery accusations and a proliferation of dark rumors of impending destruction and death. Heil's Aborigines seem to be in the middle, secure in their social orientation in being "one of us," but nonetheless wholly dependent upon the Australian state for economic subsistence. They lack, it seems, the cultural confidence of the Cree, but are not now experiencing the terrifying vertigo of transformation of the Matsigenka. Despite the widespread misunderstanding by the Australian state and its experts, they nonetheless seem able to maintain their salient senses of well-being, in Heil's account. These small-scale societies thus range in their responses to state and world from cultural bafflement, to expressions of sociocultural although not economic autonomy, to a considerable degree of cultural confidence.

As all three chapters clearly show, this sense of cultural autonomy and efficacy is directly related to informants' senses of well-being. In a small-scale society, one's cultural identity and one's sense of well-being are intrinsically linked, at least according to these accounts—a correlation that may be considerably less direct in many large-scale societies. In any case, these three ethnographic chapters trace out a fascinating set of portraits of well-being threatened and at least potentially regained.

Part Three's three chapters, set in India, China, and Japan, are based in the relation of individuals to culture and to state in three large-scale contemporary societies. Derné's chapter 6 shows how the young Indian men he interviewed found well-being not in asserting their individual desires in finding a wife, but rather in following the dictates of family in their choice of partner, in particular their fathers. This "sociocentric cultural orientation," as he labels it, does not negate individual desires--"a balance between independence and group guidance is cross-culturally necessary for people to experience well-being," he writes—but does exist as an overriding orientation among these young Indian men, one that may make assertion of one's individual desires seem terrifying, and one that global mass media, in its emphasis on romantic love, has thus far failed to shake. This orientation is one that, in Derné's account, is strikingly different from that held by middle-class Americans. His argument interestingly parallels that of Heil in chapter 4, with her informants resisting through their strong social bonds the Western individualistic norm. But it also, surprisingly, has a degree of resonance with Weisner's account of American families in chapter 11, whose members, within his familial interviews, emphasize not individual desires but rather making their families "work."

Jankowiak in chapter 7 offers a strikingly different picture of well-being from that of Derné. His Chinese informants suffered during the communist era in China in the 1980s—under such a regime, they felt no control over their lives, and sank into apathy and despair. But with the opening up of China's market economy, the ending of many governmental restrictions in daily life, and "the expansion of personal horizons," senses of well-being improved dramatically, he tells us. Jankowiak emphasizes the universal importance of a sense of individual control over one's life, in contrast to Derné's argument for an Indian sociocentric orientation as opposed to an American individualistic orientation. He also differs in emphasizing political and economic more than cultural factors in shaping the senses of well-being of his informants. Jankowiak stresses that the complex cultural roots of Chinese senses of well-being have been distorted by recent decades of totalitarian social control. His argument is not about "culture" as an encompassing value orientation, but about how an intrusive economic and political system can suppress well-being, just as its removal can cause an explosion in well-being. Derné and Jankowiak seem at odds. Their discussions with one another over the course of putting this volume together shaped the chapters each wrote, but did not fundamentally alter their different points of view, as shaped by their different ethnographic sites and what they found there.

Mathews' chapter 8 provides one way of reconciling the apparently contradictory findings of Derné and Jankowiak. Mathews explores "what makes life worth living" in Japan, through the Japanese term *ikigai,* perhaps the only everyday term in all the world's languages that refers to such a matter. He then applies this term elsewhere, examining the cultural formulations, social negotiations, and institutional channelings of "what makes life worth living" among Japanese, Americans, and Hong Kongers in comparison, to arrive at a condensed picture of the pursuit of *ikigai* in three societies. We can apply this to Derné and Jankowiak's chapters. Many of Derné's Indian informants view their natal families as their *ikigai,* as what is most important to them in their lives, while many of Jankowiak's Chinese informants seem to have had no *ikigai* during the communist years, and have discovered it with the coming of choice in their lives. For many of Derné's Indian informants, attachment to natal family is a matter of taken-for-granted cultural common sense: "cultural fate," in Mathews' term. For Jankowiak's Chinese, on the other hand, the newfound sense of control over their lives represents an escape from the oppressive weight of institutional channeling of the communist years. That oppressive weight was not experienced as cultural common sense, intrinsic to one's self, but a power extrinsic to oneself to which one had to conform, a matter not of internal culture but external institutions. Derné's informants thus reflect cultural shaping seen as intrinsic to oneself and thus to be upheld and defended, while Jankowiak's informants reflect institutional channeling seen as external to oneself and thus to be repelled—the difference, to put it far too simply, between family and state in shaping one's life.

Underlying the above analysis, it seems clear that, rather than straightforward cultural differences in different societies (i.e., "sociocentric Indians" and "individualistic Americans," as expressed in numerous earlier works of anthropology and other social sciences: for example Bellah et al.1985; Dumont 1980; Hsu 1985; Geertz 1983), we instead see human universals in the pursuit of well-being, that come to the fore differently in different societies and different social contexts but that are present in every society. Human beings need the support of, if not necessarily their families, then very definitely their human social world. Human beings also tend to seek freedom from coercive control, especially if that control is thought to be not intrinsic to oneself but externally imposed—human beings need some sense of control over and efficacy in their lives. Human beings also need a sense of life being worth living in a given society. If that is not the case, if a serious "legitimation crisis" is at hand, then a society will lose its members' allegiance in various ways, as is taking place in a range of societies today, according to Mathews, and as took place in 1980s China, by Jankowiak's account. The above formulation does not entail a functionalist theory of well-being, but it does seem plausible that there are universal aspects of individual well-being that societies everywhere must more or less fulfill, as depicted by the three chapters in this section.

The three chapters in Part Four offer new directions, exploring three particular aspects of well-being not often considered in anthropological research, and offer different frameworks enabling cross-cultural comparison.

Clark in chapter 9 explores well-being through physical pleasure and its cultural structuring. This is a neglected aspect of well-being, perhaps because it is so hard to describe, yet it is clearly universal and also fundamentally culturally shaped. Bathing can be understood through the analytical conjunction of three elements, Clark tells us: its setting, "the equipment of the mundane bath necessary for a pleasurable experience"; its activity, the specific sequence of events necessary in order to experience the bath in a Japanese context; and the array of cultural meanings given to the experience of the bath, including cleanliness/ purity, health/vigor, and Japanese identity itself.

Hollan in chapter 10 considers the subjective experience of the "self-scape." Well-being, although indubitably shaped by one's sociocultural world, is inherently individual, Hollan argues. Well-being is a matter of how well one's mind/body is felt to fit within one's physical and social world, and is never static but rather is in dynamic flux. Hollan illustrates this through his intimate portrait of a typical day in the life of the Toraja man Nene'na Tandi, a life that is contrasted between the security of home and family and the tension of being outside, especially in passage to his gardens and rice fields, where he is susceptible to the magic of enemies. Nene'na Tandi's well-being is shaped both positively and negatively by his dreams and encounters in the spirit world.

Weisner, in chapter 11, takes a different approach than Hollan, and indeed all the other chapters in this book. Although he does interview individuals, he does so only within the family unit. He thus in effect leaves aside the individual as a unit of analysis, to examine families, and the efforts of families with children with disabilities to maintain sustainable routines—a key component of well-being, in his view, which he defines as "engaged participation in everyday cultural activities that are deemed desirable by a community." Weisner's chapter alone among the ethnographic chapters of this volume offers a specific universal definition of well-being. His turn away from the individual, to analyze the "social construction of well-being," separates well-being from individual consciousness alone, showing not its individual but its collective basis. Only Weisner's research among that reported in this book uses both survey instruments and ethnographic interviews taking place over more than a decade to gauge how these families are coping; he alone is pursuing the combination of survey research and ethnography advocated by Colby.

These analyses tackle well-being in fundamentally different ways, using different analytical foci; they also each offer specific frameworks for the comparison of well-being across a range of different societies. Clark, because he deals with pleasure, which is all but ineffable since we cannot fully experience another's pleasure as he or she feels it, analyzes pleasure largely apart from individual consciousness, examining settings, activities, and cultural meanings instead, and wonders whether those outside the Japanese cultural nexus can ever fully understand Japanese pleasure as Japanese can. Hollan, expressing no such doubt, daringly examines the phenomenological experience of a single individual. He enters directly into the mind of his informant, to portray his daily experiences in all their intimacy. The advantage of this strategy is that it enables us, more than in any other chapter of this book, to see the world through the mind of another, in an extraordinarily close portrayal of what the shifting gradients of well-being feel like for a particular Toraja man. But we may ask, how does Hollan know this? Hollan knows of Nene'na Tandi's experience because he asked him about it in extensive interviewing—but can the words of another person fully convey the experience of that person? To what extent is Nene'na Tandi's experience finally Hollan's imaginative reconstruction, a second-hand account that cannot portray first-hand experience? No other anthropologist in this volume is willing to take this analytic tack, and Mathews in chapter 8 specifically repudiates it; and yet, if well-being is to be fully understood in its subjective basis, its most fundamental reality as discussed in our introduction, then perhaps this step is not only allowable but necessary—even if problematic.[2]

Weisner takes an altogether different approach, eschewing the analysis of individuals except as members of families; we know those whom he interviews only as members of families. How many of the parents among his informants hold private dreams of escape from their familial bonds? And how do the developmentally delayed children in these families themselves feel about the lives and social worlds into which they have been born? We cannot know this about his informants from his chapter. Nonetheless, Weisner's analysis is important in its intentional neglect of the individual except in the context of family. Why, indeed, should the autonomous individual be privileged, given the fact that we all live within social networks? Derné in chapter 6 and Heil in chapter 4 critique American and Western individualistic assumptions; Weisner, in his chapter, methodologically moves beyond those assumptions. This is a daring move indeed—in a sense the exact opposite of

Hollan's move—but not without potential analytical costs in its leaving aside the examination of "selfish" individual motivations.

All these different research strategies have their lacunae, yet all show great promise in enabling the anthropological comparison of aspects of well-being down different methodological and epistemological lines. The last four chapters of this book offer specific theoretical and methodological analytical tools that seem eminently practicable cross-culturally—even if they are all necessarily partial, as we will now discuss.

Well-Being and Societal Comparison

The ethnographic chapters of this book can be criticized on several grounds. One ground—referring not simply to these chapters alone, but to anthropology as a whole today—is the view of culture that these chapters present. To what extent are people today cocooned within discrete cultures? Perhaps less than some of these chapters imply. Whether they are Australian Aborigine, Cree, Chinese, Japanese, or American, people today are exposed to a range of different influences: they are a part of an array of different communities, to varying degrees, and have access to a range of information and identities beyond those explicitly proffered by their own societies. To some extent at least, well-being among individuals in a given society cannot be fully understood without taking into account these different influences.

Related to this, many of this book's chapters do not sufficiently emphasize the diversity of senses of well-being within the societies they describe, a diversity refracted through social class, age, and especially gender. We might also ask to what extent the people portrayed in these ethnographic chapters are controlled by their societies and cultures and to what extent they have a degree of individual agency. Clearly they do have some degree of individual agency, but this is only implicitly visible in some of this book's ethnographic chapters. Well-being is certainly shaped by social structure and culture, but also by individual past experience and present choice; but except in Hollan's chapter 10 and Mathews' chapter 8, this is not much emphasized. These criticisms are not directed primarily at this book's chapters, but at anthropological treatments of culture in general, which seem undeveloped despite many recent criticisms (for example, Brightman 1995; Mathews 2000). However, these criticisms need to be addressed in order for anthropology to be able to deal with well-being in all its complexity. Colby's concept of "self-world" rather than "culture" as a unit of analysis, as discussed in chapter 2, seems a good place to start.

Turning now to well-being itself, as is readily apparent from the preceding discussion, well-being is not treated by anthropologists as a single entity. Rather, the different anthropological analyses in this book focus on different aspects of well-being. We see in the book's chapters fundamentally discrepant forms of analysis, discrepancies based on the societies being studied and also on the particular aspects of well-being that are being examined.

These analytic discrepancies are ultimately due to the nature of anthropology as a discipline. As we saw in the introduction, other disciplines look at well-being in very specific ways. Economists and policy specialists may explore well-being through statistical measures such as per capita income and life expectancy, while psychologists may measure well-being through surveys asking people to rate their satisfaction with life on a numerical scale. These measures themselves in effect define what well-being is. However, anthropology as a discipline is far more diverse. Accordingly, the chapters of this book have very different approaches to well-being. The biggest reason for this diversity is that anthropologists tend to study topics that are of particular salience to their informants, as the chapters earlier discussed so richly reveal. Every ethnographic chapter in this book investigates in different ways "the native's point of view," in Malinowski's words forming an epigraph to Thin's chapter, which is, according to most anthropologists today, the essence of anthropological investigation.

The upshot of this situation is the opposite of that which pertains to disciplines such as psychology and economics. If psychology and economics allow for easy comparability of well-being analyzed shallowly—by assuming, in research design and measurement, common conceptions of well-being for everyone—anthropology allows for difficult comparability of well-being analyzed deeply. An unkind critic might say that the anthropological investigations of well-being portrayed in this book are like the blind men and the elephant: each investigator takes a different approach, analyzing a different aspect of well-being, and conceiving of well-being in its particular light. But a broader view would be that in focusing on particular issues of particular importance in given societies, these anthropologists are showing that the one-size-fits-all model of well-being held by psychologists and economists is insufficient to understand well-being in particular societies, where very particular concerns and formulations hold sway. Detailed knowledge of a given society's particularity is absolutely essential if we are to understand well-being in that society.

This is revealed by every ethnographic chapter in this book. To give just a few examples, one cannot understand well-being among the Matsigenka unless one understands numerous interrelated cultural strands in their recent past and present. For example, the role of the evangelical protestant church among the Matsigenka, the place of shamanism in Matsigenka lives, the role of curers in their ethnomedical system, the classificatory kinship system they use and its effect in leading many people in the community to assume quasi-parental roles in childrearing, and the cultural threat Matsigenka face before the onslaught of oil companies such as Plus Petrol—all of this very particular ethnographic data has a direct effect on Matsigenka well-being. One cannot understand well-being in China today without understanding cultural traditions striving to link body and mind together into spiritual wholeness, and the traditional Chinese sense of "having been born to be happy" as attained through one's own proactive behavior; the Chinese communist social organization of work units and its far-reaching effects on individuals' daily life; the Cultural Revolution and its subsequent effects on senses of the legitimacy of the communist state; and the complex Chinese transition from communist state to capitalist market and its effects on people's senses of their lives. One cannot understand well-being in Japan today without understanding positive Japanese attitudes towards physical pleasure, including the subtle nuances of the various overlapping Japanese terms used to connote enjoyment, and the rituals of everyday bathing, whether in one's home or in large public bathing facilities. One cannot understand Japanese well-being without understanding the complex and contradictory array of meanings given to a term such as *ikigai*, that which makes one's life worth living; and one cannot understand Japanese well-being as a whole without considering numerous other areas of Japanese life as well, from the economic downturn of the past fifteen years, to the changing structure of Japanese gender roles, to Japanese perceptions of foreign countries and the world beyond Japan. In every one of these cases, statistical measures of well-being would in and of themselves be grossly inadequate. We must understand in detail the ethnographic context, as these chapters portray, to be able to understand well-being in these societies.

This is what anthropology can offer—a sociocultural contextualizing that can enable us to make sense of how people in different societies feel about their lives. If this alone is what anthropology can provide the study of well-being, then anthropology will have made a great contribution—this alone makes this book worth reading and worth writing, we believe. But for anthropology to provide something more, we must move beyond ethnographic description alone, to examine comparison: what kinds of anthropological comparison of well-being are possible?

The first two chapters of this book advocate comparisons that are too sweeping to be followed by most of the ethnographic chapters of this book. But other kinds of comparison are more limited, and thus more practicable. Part Two's comparisons of small-scale societies are effective because (1) these societies can be described with a degree of comprehensiveness by a single anthropologist; (2) cultural identity and well-being are closely linked in these societies, as we have discussed, enabling discussions of well-being to take place in the context of culture and cultural identity; and (3) these societies, although scattered across the globe, share considerable commonality, as cultural groups struggling to maintain themselves against the pressures and predations of state and world. Indeed, one can envision a volume on well-being in small-scale societies that would amplify the themes of these three chapters. Such a book could offer useful insights about sustaining well-being among small-scale societies across the globe in a nationalizing, globalizing world.

Effective comparison becomes more difficult when the analytical focus is societies not of hundreds or thousands of people, but millions or hundreds of millions. Derné and Jankowiak in Part Three generalize about India and China, but this is to some extent problematic, given the fact that they each had a few dozen informants. Indian sociocentrism and Chinese rejoicing at freedom from state control are broadly shared cultural values in the two societies, but with many nuances that we cannot see—these authors lacked the space in their brief chapters to fully trace out these nuances. The problem of representation can be partially overcome by using mass media articles as well as statistical data from the society being examined, to correlate one's small-scale findings with broader forms of information. One can envision a book-length comparison of well-being in India and China, using the kind of close ethnographic research conducted in these two chapters as well as other kinds of data, examining through individual accounts the well-being of these two societies that are the key to the world's economic future. For that matter, one could also ethnographically examine the well-being of citizens among leading capitalist societies today—Western European nations, Japan, and the United States—to better understand how state and corporate policies impact upon everyday lives, and to comprehend comparative senses of happiness among those who live in these different societies. What are the costs and benefits of each form of capitalism to the lives and dreams of these different societies' members? What varieties of contemporary capitalism—if any—might be most conducive to a fuller human existence? Anthropology needs a latter-day Max

Weber to make such a comparison, but perhaps that day will not be long in coming.

The last four chapters of the book leave aside these universal comparisons, to instead offer comparison on much more specific grounds. None of these methods as set forth in these chapters applies to well-being at large, but rather, to particular aspects of well-being—well-being considered from a particular angle. But these more focused frames of enquiry offer comparison that is ethnographically rigorous, and that thus can be highly useful—even if, as we've seen, these frames of enquiry are focused on more fine-grained types of comparison than that of well-being at large.

We have seen how the stumbling block in anthropological analyses of well-being is that, because of their emphasis on "the native's point of view," many anthropologists, including the ethnographic chapter-writers of this book, do not emphasize well-being as a whole, which is an experience-far concept, foreign to most of the people that anthropologists investigate. Rather, they examine specific angles on and aspects of well-being that reflect the concerns of the people they are studying. This is as it should be: if cultural anthropology is not driven by the concerns of the people it studies, then it loses its raison d'être. But this also removes anthropology from direct investigation into well-being, which is on one level no more than an awkward and technical English-language locution, but on another level a concern of everyone on the planet. Happiness may be pursued in multiple ways and down multiple paths, but it is pursued everywhere. One way to navigate around this problem is to broadly map out well-being, and then examine where our chapters fit within its purview.

Considering all that we have explored concerning well-being in this book's chapters, it seems that we may divide well-being into four experiential dimensions. Three of these dimensions parallel the realms for a theory of well-being set forth by Colby in his chapter 2; the fourth is our own addition. There is a physical dimension of well-being, involving how individuals conceive, perceive, and experience their bodies in the world. There is an interpersonal dimension of well-being, involving how individuals conceive, perceive, and experience their relation with others. There is an existential dimension to well-being, involving how individuals comprehend the values and meanings of their lives. These three dimensions are structured by a fourth dimension, involving how national institutions and global forces shape how well-being is conceived, perceived, and experienced among individuals in different societies. All of these dimensions are perceived through a prism of culture, which shapes the apprehension of all four dimensions in any given society.

Our argument is that anthropologists may investigate these different dimensions of well-being, and societies may be compared as to where they fit within these different dimensions of well-being. Of course, just as comparison of well-being as a whole is often difficult across societies, so too comparison within these specific dimensions, not least because different societies culturally slice up these different dimensions in different ways. Nonetheless, we argue that by providing a specific analytic focus on a particular dimension of well-being rather than on the concept as a whole in all its breadth, we have the basis for a cross-cultural comparative schema of well-being, through which aspects of well-being within particular societies can be more fully analyzed and understood.

Let us go over each of these dimensions in turn, as they relate to the book's ethnographic chapters. Human beings of all societies have conceptions of and experience of pleasure (short-term physical well-being) and health (long-term physical well-being). This is due to the biological bases of well-being that Colby discusses in chapter 2, biological bases that are culturally shaped to a very large degree. Clark's chapter 9, emphasizing the exquisite culturally shaped pleasures of the Japanese bath, convincingly shows the mixture of universal and cultural aspects of pleasure. This is no doubt true for a vast range of physical pleasures, from smoking hookahs to drinking wine to jogging. As for health, Izquierdo's chapter 3 and Heil's chapter 4 both are at pains to demonstrate that physical health and social and societal well-being are fundamentally different. They are reacting against the assumption, so prevalent in Western medical and public-health discourses, that physical health and well-being are the same thing; in the realm of well-being, the social and interpersonal overrides the physical, they are both saying.

Of the chapters in this book, only Clark's chapter 9 devotes itself to the physical dimension of well-being, but his chapter, as well as every other ethnographic chapter in this book, also is rooted in the interpersonal dimension of well-being. Human beings of all societies are fundamentally dependent on others for survival: a physical dependence, but more—a social dependence, as exemplified by language. Different societies culturally emphasize interpersonal dependence to different degrees; Heil in chapter 4 and Derné in chapter 6 show us societies that particularly emphasize reliance on one's social world, whereas Jankowiak in chapter 7 emphasizes individual liberation from sociopolitical constraints. But in all this book's chapters, the social/interpersonal is the most pivotal realm of well-being. This is what all the book's ethnographic chapters show, even those, such as Hollan's chapter 10, that focus resolutely on individual consciousness. Ethnography, in its emphasis on the depiction of social life through participant-observation and interviewing, is particularly well suited to illustrate the subtleties of this dimension of well-being. This dimension of well-being is anthropology's home, so to speak. But interestingly, apart for Weisner's chapter 11 with its focus on families, interpersonal well-being is analyzed in most of this book's chapters through individuals. Weisner's chapter, uniquely in this book, offers a means of getting at well-being not through the individual but through the interpersonal dimension.

As cultural beings, human beings seek to explain our lives—why we are alive and what our lives mean. This is true in every society, albeit in different culturally shaped forms (Becker 1971), ranging from myths told around a campfire, to incantations of priests or imams, to religious scriptures, to Hollywood and Bollywood movies. This is the existential dimension of well-being. Most of the chapters in this book do not directly focus on this dimension. Izquierdo (chapter 3) and Hollan (chapter 10) both touch upon the existential realm, as do, more indirectly through their informants' comments, Derné (chapter 6) and Jankowiak (chapter 7), but the only chapter that makes the existential dimension its central concern is that of Mathews (chapter 8). This is largely because Mathews stumbled across the Japanese term *ikigai*, "what makes life worth living," a concept that exists in prosaic everyday language apparently only in Japanese. It may be that the existential dimension is a comparatively difficult aspect of well-being to ethnographically explore, simply in that people don't tend to talk about it readily with others, and many societies have, outside of religious ceremonies, relatively few cultural avenues in which it may be directly explored.

Finally, there is the dimension of national institutions and global forces, readily apparent in most of the ethnographic chapters of this book. Only the chapters of Part Four do not much discuss this dimension, largely because all three of these chapters are setting forth new approaches and methodologies for the study of well-being, and thus lack the space to cover this dimension. However, undoubtedly it affects the informants in these chapters, from government regulations concerning baths in Japan to welfare and educational provisions for developmentally delayed children in the United States. For the small-scale societies depicted in Part Two, the impact of nation and world is absolutely essential—this is exactly what is threatening these societies' survival. For the large-scale societies depicted in Part Three as well, national policies and globalization are inescapable, as these chapters all explore.

We thus see that the interpersonal dimension and the national/global dimension of well-being are most examined in our ethnographic chapters, while the physical dimension and the existential dimension are least examined. This reflects the discipline of anthropology as a whole, in which human social life in all its forms, as impacted by national and global forces, is at the mainstream of anthropological research, and the physical and existential realms of inquiry are treated less frequently, in the side currents and eddies of the discipline. These mainstream areas of inquiry are where the ethnographic contribution to the study of well-being is likely to be fullest, but all four of these dimensions are amenable to anthropological inquiry. Anthropology students interested in well-being and happiness who are looking for new areas of inquiry might consider the physical and the existential dimensions for their research. These are areas that, not just in this book but in anthropology as a whole, are comparatively under-researched. Anthropologists may not seek to make well-being per se the central focus of their research, for the reasons discussed earlier, but rather focus on a central issue of concern for those they are ethnographically investigating. Nonetheless, by being aware of well-being and what its cross-cultural meanings and implications are, anthropologists will be far better situated to place their particular ethnographic work within a larger field: that of the investigation of human happiness in all its enculturated forms.

And indeed, why not embark upon such an investigative path? In an increasingly globalized world, when we are all ever more in each other's faces and lives, ethnographically informed "soft comparison" of societies as to well-being becomes increasingly plausible, and increasingly necessary. Richard Shweder has written that, to the question, "Which society is the best place to raise children?" he would answer as follows: "There is no single best place to be raised. ... But one of the really good places to be raised is any place where you learn that there is no single best place to be raised. ... I call that place postmodern humanism, or the view from manywheres" (2003, 1–2). We who edit this book largely agree with this view. There are value judgments to be made about the societies described in this book. Jankowiak's Chinese do indeed appear far happier today, by his account, than twenty-five years ago, when they were under state totalitarian control. Adelson's Cree do indeed appear to be more secure in their well-being than Izquierdo's Matsigenka. In a broader sense, certainly well-being is more easily attainable for many people today in Japan or the United States or China than in Iraq or Gaza or the Darfur region of the Sudan, or other societies wracked by violence and poverty. But beyond these broad parameters, we cannot make firm judgments, but must investigate and celebrate diversity:

there are indeed multiple pursuits of happiness. One of the most positive things about the world today is that we can increasingly come to understand one another's pursuits in all their multiplicity, adding them to the sum of knowledge we have about how to live. This has been the purpose of this book: to portray and analyze societies within the panorama of human well-beings, and thus arrive at a fuller understanding of the multiple ways in which we might live and live well. And who knows—perhaps through the anthropological analysis of well-being, as presented in this book's pages, we might ourselves learn to live better and more happily.

Notes

1. This is all the more the case given the biological basis of well-being that Colby stresses, indicating a common human basis for the measurement of well-being. Many anthropologists resist this; but see Cronk 1999 and more unpalatably, Wilson 1998, for arguments as to links of the cultural to the biological in human endeavors.
2. This is problematic because of the fundamental epistemological difficulties involved in entering the mind of another human being. See Harris 1989 for a skeptical view of "entering the mind of another" in anthropology; see Schutz 1970 and Cohen 1994 for somewhat more sympathetic views.

References

Becker, Ernest. 1971. *The Birth and Death of Meaning: An Interdisciplinary Perspective On the Problem of Man*. 2nd ed. New York: The Free Press.
Bellah, Robert N., Richard Madsen, William M. Sullivan, Ann Swidler, and Steven M. Tipton. 1985. *Habits of the Heart: Individualism and Commitment in American Life*. New York: Harper and Row.
Brightman, Robert. 1995. "Forget Culture: Replacement, Transcendence, Relexification." *Cultural Anthropology* 10 (4): 509–46.
Cohen, Anthony P. 1994. *Self-Consciousness: An Alternative Anthropology of Identity*. London: Routledge.
Cronk, Lee. 1999. *That Complex Whole: Culture and the Evolution of Human Behavior*. Boulder, CO: Westview Press.
Dumont, Louis. 1980. *Homo Hierarchicus: The Caste System and Its Implications*. Chicago: University of Chicago Press.
Geertz, Clifford. 1983. "'From the Native's Point of View': On the Nature of Anthropological Understanding." In *Local Knowledge: Further Essays in Anthropological Understanding*. New York: Basic Books.
Harris, Grace Gredys. 1989. "Concepts of Individual, Self, and Person in Description and Analysis." *American Anthropologist* 91 (3): 599–612.

Hatch, Elvin. 1983. *Culture and Morality: The Relativity of Values in Anthropology.* New York: Columbia University Press.

Hsu, Francis L. K. 1985. "The Self in Cross-cultural Perspective." In *Culture and Self: Asian and Western Perspectives,* ed. A. Marsella, G. DeVos, and F. L. K. Hsu. New York: Tavistock Publications.

Mathews, Gordon. 2000. *Global Culture/Individual Identity: Searching for Home in the Cultural Supermarket.* London: Routledge.

Scheper-Hughes, Nancy. 1995. "The Primacy of the Ethical: Propositions for a Militant Anthropology." *Current Anthropology* 36 (3): 409–20.

Schutz, Alfred. 1970. *On Phenomenology and Social Relations,* ed. R. Wagner. Chicago: University of Chicago Press.

Shweder, Richard A. 2003. "Introduction: Anti-Postculturalism (or, the View from Manywheres)." In *Why Do Men Barbecue?: Recipes for Cultural Psychology.* Cambridge, MA: Harvard University Press.

Wilson, E. O. 1998. *Consilience: The Unity of Knowledge.* New York: Vintage Books.

Index

Lightning Source UK Ltd.
Milton Keynes UK
UKOW04f2102010916

281914UK00001B/96/P